THE CLASSIC WORK THAT HAS BEEN AN ESSENTIAL
REFERENCE FOR THOUSANDS OF ANOREXICS, THEIR
FAMILIES, AND THEIR MEDICAL PRACTITIONERS.

TREATING AND OVERCOMING
ANOREXIA NERVOSA

Because of new changes in the health care system that
shortens hospital stays and doesn't fully cover day programs
with insurance, more of the responsibility for care of the
anorexic falls on parents or partners. This comprehensive
guide by Steven Levenkron, one of America's top specialists,
will make that emotionally difficult job easier by providing
specific guidance in what to expect, what to do, and how to
really help. Written in plain English, using the cases of real
people, fully indexed, and supplying detailed information on
hospitalization and support groups, this is the reference
work every family touched by this heartbreaking disorder
must have.

* * *

"One of the most lucid and detailed accounts to be found
anywhere of the theory and techniques of psychotherapeu-
tic work with people afflicted with anorexia nervosa."
—Jack L. Katz, M.D.,
Chairman of the Department of Psychology,
North Shore University Hospital

Please turn the page for more expert endorsements . . .

"This book should be compulsory reading for families of anorexic patients as well as for all professionals who deal with them."

—Virginia E. Pomeranz, M.D., co-author,
The Mother's and Father's Medical Encyclopedia

"There is refreshing wisdom in this book; Levenkron offers authentic hope to anorexics, to their families, and to psychotherapists as well. This work is a major advance to the theory and treatment of anorexia."

—Barnard Landis, Ph.D.,
Clinical Associate Professor,
Cornell University Medical College

"With clarity and insightfulness, Steve Levenkron demonstrates why conventional psychotherapeutic methods are often not effective."

—Vivian Meehan, President,
National Association of Anorexia and
Associated Disorders (ANAD)

ABOUT THE AUTHOR

STEVEN LEVENKRON has treated anorexia nervosa since 1970 as part of his full-time psychotherapy practice in New York City. He has held positions in many prominent hospitals in the New York metropolitan area, among them clinical consultant at Montefiore Hospital and Medical Center, clinical consultant at the Center for the Study of Anorexia and Bulimia in New York City, adjunct director at the Eating Disorder Service at Four Winds Psychiatric Hospital in Westchester, N.Y., and currently he is a member of the advisory board of the National Association of Anorexia and Associated Disorders (ANAD) in Highland Park, Illinois.

His 1978 novel, *The Best Little Girl in the World*, made into a top-rated ABC-TV movie of the week in 1981, brought him international recognition as an authority on anorexia nervosa. His 1991 book, *Obsessive-Compulsive Disorders*, brought him recognition in a second but related disorder.

Steven Levenkron lives in New York with his family.

Also by Steven Levenkron

The Best Little Girl in the World
Obsessive-Compulsive Disorders

Published by
WARNERBOOKS

TREATING AND OVERCOMING
ANOREXIA NERVOSA

STEVEN LEVENKRON

WARNER BOOKS

A Time Warner Company

This book is not intended as a substitute for medical advice. The reader should regularly consult a physician or health care professional in matters relating to health and particulary in respect to any symptoms which may require diagnosis or medical attention.

If you purchase this book without a cover you should be aware that this book may have been stolen property and reported as "unsold and destroyed" to the publisher. In such case neither the author nor the publisher has received any payment for this "stripped book."

For my wife
Abby
and my daughters
Rachel and Gabrielle

Acknowledgments

My thanks go to Dr. Virginia Pomeranz for her encouragement in my psychotherapeutic endeavors. I am grateful to the staff of New York's Montefiore Hospital and Medical Center: to Dr. Preston Zucker for his personal and professional support as well as for his sensitive and vital care for those patients who had to be hospitalized; to Dr. Michael I. Cohen, chairman of the Department of Pediatrics at Montefiore and at the Albert Einstein College of Medicine for the trust he had in the team approach; to Dr. Kenneth Schoenberg for the headaches he puts up with; to Dr. Jack Katz in the Department of Psychiatry for making available his psychopharmacological knowledge and understanding; to Dr. Scott Boley, chairman of the Department of Pediatric Surgery; and to Drs. Sylvain Kleinhaus and Michael Sheran, who had daily responsibility for the surgically implanted catheters that saved the lives of many patients over the last five years. Thanks also to Dr. Everett Dulit for his problem-solving advice, and to the nursing staff at North-West Six for their understanding help to my patients. Also thanks to Carole Sharin for her thoughtful editing and typing skills in the preparation of this manuscript. My thanks also to Susanne Kirk for her personable and efficient help in editing the manuscript and steering it into production.

Contents

Foreword

Several years ago, Steven Levenkron and I found ourselves in a strange situation. We had patients with anorexia nervosa being referred to us from all parts of the country. We had a major teaching hospital with extensive research investment in anorexia willing to care for these patients. But we lacked therapists willing or able to treat anorexics. In an attempt to educate capable therapists in the treatment of anorexics, we organized a conference in New York City and sent out more than two thousand invitations through mailing lists supplied by local psychotherapeutic societies in New York, New Jersey, and Connecticut. Only seven replies were returned.

I have found two recurrent reasons why so few therapists treat anorexics: these patients are time consuming and demanding, and classic psychotherapy often does not work. Failure is indeed frightening in a major disease with a 10 to 15 percent mortality rate. That usual methods of treatment often fail is not surprising. The disease crosses standard lines of psychiatric classification—aspects of body image and feelings about food and eating seem delusional, while the patient in every other way seems coherent, logical, and even overachieving.

Steven Levenkron's book attempts to encourage more psychotherapists to treat anorexia nervosa. I have seen the "nurturant authoritative psychotherapy" that is discussed in this book work, but I will leave it to the behavioral scholars to argue its merits and faults and to refine it.

I am a pediatric gastroenterologist rather than a psychiatrist. I became involved in the treatment of anorexia when called upon by several psychotherapists, including the author, to utilize total parenteral nutrition as a life-saving medical therapy in severe anorexics. The anorexia nervosa treatment unit of the Division of Adolescent Medicine at Montefiore Hospital and Medical Center in New York City developed out of this experience.

One has only to look at pictures of the blank, vacant stares in the faces of starving people throughout the world to realize that an anorexic cannot think clearly enough to climb out of the abyss of a self-imposed starvation. A severely starved patient must receive adequate nutrition before any progress in psychotherapy can take place. The psychotherapist is not trained or skilled in nutritional assessment, nor does he or she have to be. The therapist needs a second part of the "team," a physician who says to the patient, "Your therapist is in charge of your head; I am in charge of your body. He will get you well; I will keep you alive while he is doing it."

The medical doctor must make clear to the patient that he is her doctor and not an extension of her parents. He, like the therapist, must develop the patient's imperturbable faith in him. He should divorce himself from the parents by dealing with the patient alone, never disclosing anything but general information to parents, especially not divulging actual weights unless explicitly allowed by the patient.

Good communication between the therapist and the medical doctor is also essential. Progress in increasing dietary intake frequently adds to anxieties. Weekly communication between professionals can often prevent a crisis or warn of impending problems. Many anorexics try to play the physician against the therapist or vice versa, but if the doctor and therapist are working well together they can prevent this situation and the regression that inevitably accompanies it.

Anorexia nervosa is a formidable disease of epidemic proportions currently affecting over 3 percent of our female college population. As with any formidable disease, early diagnosis and appropriate treatment will result in a significant cure rate. To combat this epidemic we need an army of experienced psychotherapists with medical support, in addition to the continuing research that looks for the ultimate in medical care, prevention.

I hope this book and others like it will help form the basic training manual of that army.

Preston Zucker, M.D.
ASSOCIATE CLINICAL PROFESSOR OF PEDIATRICS
MONTEFIORE HOSPITAL AND MEDICAL CENTER
ALBERT EINSTEIN COLLEGE OF MEDICINE

INTRODUCTION TO THE REVISED EDITION
by Steven Levenkron

Twenty years ago *anorexia nervosa* was an esoteric term used by a small group of physicians and therapists who began to see a number of emaciated young girls as patients. Over the years the number of diagnosed anorexic patients has increased at an alarming rate as professionals are better informed in identifying victims of anorexia nervosa. In fact, one out of 250 teenage girls succumbs to the disorder for the sake of losing a few pounds. The disorder will prove fatal to 9% of its victims. Of those lucky enough to undergo treatment, less than half will recover completely.

The medical community and families of anorexics are up against a stubborn enemy. Furthermore, the recent changes in the health care system available to anorexics have resulted in shorter hospital treatment time and have shifted more responsibility for the treatment and care of patients to less-experienced physicians and psychotherapists. More of the financial and emotional burden will also fall on families of the victims.

There have been three major areas of change in the treatment of anorexia nervosa since the original publication of TREATING AND OVERCOMING ANOREXIA NERVOSA:

—Changes in the health care system
—Introduction of antidepressants in the treatment of AN
—Financial and emotional impact on families of anorexics

First, we must take a closer look at the changes in

health care. These changes restrict hospital stay to four weeks, even though in most cases it takes eight to nine weeks of hospital stay to stabilize weight loss in the critical stages of anorexia nervosa and assure that the patient is out of danger. During this stage the hospital provides round-the-clock supervision of eating, drinking, and eliminating processes. To the patient this supervision is an unwanted intrusion, but after a week or so the patient usually begins to adjust to the supportive nature of her caretaking environment.

Treatment is not limited to bringing weight to desirable levels. Correcting unhealthy eating patterns, encouraging healthy elimination practices, and warning the patient about laxative abuse and vomiting are also addressed. A good therapist will also discourage excessive exercise practices. Above and beyond the visible, physical damages remain the invisible issues of trust, dependency, rigidity, intimacy, self-esteem, and identity.

It is during this time she begins to use the hospital staff and other patients as buffers against the grip of her anorexic behavior. In an effective treatment she will share her thoughts with others; she will listen, observe, and feel less alone, thus becoming part of a group therapy process that will *slowly* reduce her sense of emotional isolation. I emphasize that this process takes time, often months, to be effective.

In addition to participating and connecting with other members in her group therapy, an alliance or trust with an individual therapist is necessary. Any "surrender" of disordered eating behavior must be done within a positive patient/therapist climate. Without this positive relationship, the patient merely feels coerced out of her security system (anorexia), and will "cooperate" in order to escape her captors. After hospital discharge she will "get even" with those who coerced her by losing the weight "they" put on her.

Another important component in the slow process of rebuilding the life of the anorexic is the role of the family. Family therapy is an essential element during hospital treatment, to build positive family dynamics and replace the hospital climate of support and trust upon the patient's discharge. The family usually joins its own therapy group, which we call multifamily therapy. In this supportive setting, parents and siblings of the patient talk to others facing the same conflicts and problems.

Every psychiatric hospital is required to develop discharge plans to assure continuity of care. Most hospital staffs are aware of the shortcomings of early discharge, and some provide full-time day programs to assure such continuity. Day programs are expensive, and again insurance payments cover only an additional three-week period.

The key issue to remember, in this age of psychiatric health insurance reimbursement that demands cure in twenty sessions or less, is that people take many years to form their personalities, disordered or not. Time—therapeutic time—is still the great healer. It can't be rushed.

A major improvement in the treatment picture is the use of new medications available to the public through their physicians and psychiatrists, especially those specializing in pharmacology related to psychiatric disorders. One problem: the public has mixed feelings about medications that affect our thoughts and emotions.

Today we are far from understanding how certain changes in brain chemistry affect emotionally disordered behavior. Some researchers and clinicians claim that each disorder is a separate disease entity and requires its own particular medication. Other clinicians see disorders as defense mechanisms developed as an attempted solution to mental pain stemming from a combination of anxiety and depression. Even this second group of clinicians differ on whether the disorder is purely hereditary although chemical in nature, or stems from the individual's life experience both past and present. What are the implications if we use chemicals to correct feelings that are reactions to our lives rather than hereditary chemical imbalances? Are we creating "legalized junkies"? On the other hand, what if we continue to hold on to the concept of mental, emotional, and spiritual purity by refusing to prescribe this medication, thus sentencing many to unhappy and unproductive lives?

Presently there are few if any diagnostic measurement tools to assure us whether a disorder is caused by someone's job, family, upbringing, or a chemical imbalance. The question of whether lives change brain chemistry, or whether brain chemistry is solely hereditary, further complicates the issue.

We come now to the issue of the use of new medications that began with the introduction of Prozac in 1988. Prozac proved so effective that other medications producing similar effects were quickly introduced. At the time of this writing, other serotonin re-uptake inhibitors include (in order of market introduction): Zoloft, Paxil, Effexor, and Luvox.

Prescribing the proper medication is an educated guess on the part of the prescribing physician. Family and medical history, and variety and intensity of symptoms are all criteria in making the choice. What makes these new medications preferable to the older antidepressants is the relative absence of dangerous side-effects. Any side-effects are more annoying and uncomfortable than dangerous. This has encouraged physicians to prescribe them more liberally.

There is no test for fluid or tissue analysis to determine which drugs might be most helpful with the least side-effects; the prescriber and patient must simply hope for the best. The end results can range from no effect at all to what appears to be a miraculous change in feelings, thoughts, and behaviors. The duration of these positive effects can be short-term or permanent (as long as one continues to take the medication). None of these medications has been on the market long enough to determine long-term effects to the brain or body. Permanent side-effects that continue after the medication is discontinued have not been noted. The patients who benefit the most from this new group of medications are those who suffer from mild to moderate depression, accompanied by anxiety and obsessiveness.

Unfortunately, the pharmaceutical industry has labelled this group of drugs "antidepressants." There is a stigma attached to one's taking an antidepressant. If we had only referred to them by function, such as "serotonin re-uptake inhibitors," or something akin to vitamins, it would produce less conflict, resistance, and shame among those who benefit from them.

The third major area of change, and perhaps the one with the most lasting effects on both families and victims of anorexia nervosa, is the role of the family in the recovery process—in financial and emotional terms.

First-time readers of this volume seeking information will find a general profile of the illness, its victims, and their families. Parents, husbands, and partners will be guided to look at the implications of their responses to the victims: how words, voice, tone, and feelings for each other affect them. A no-fault attitude toward the anorexic they love and want to help is essential. In the text they will find clues, hints, and guidelines to analyze and change these relationships that aggravate the illness and separate the anorexic from those who love her. Improving the ability to love and form healthy attachments is vital to recovery. This is not an intellectual process. Insights are useful only when they are consistent and supported with love and appropriate actions.

If you are a parent of more than one child you know that your style of love may work for all but *one* of your children. I have had parents say to me, "I only have one unhealthy child. All the rest are fine." The implication here is that it must be the child's defect that makes her ill. While the parent's usual style of expressing love works for the other child (children), this *one* needs something different. Whether the reason is due to birth order (siblings have a way of affecting each other as they compete for parental approval), chemical or genetic differences, differences in intelligence skills and aptitudes, no two children respond to parental love in exactly the same way. Many parents can take their parenting style so personally that they lose sight of the fact that parental love must meet different emotional needs in each child. They identify their parenting styles as their souls; they see any adjustments as rejection of their core selves. Today in family therapy we talk about family systems; by looking at the family system we shift some of the focus and blame off parents. Parents have to detach their parenting styles from their personal identities to make them more suitable to the needs of the child with psychological disorders or the child who is showing hints and signs that may lead to these disorders.

Parent-child relationships are often loaded with fear, anger, attachment, neediness, impatience, fatigue, love, and hatred. Add divorce and remarriage to the mix and the relationship becomes even more complex. When we examine these elements and their effects on parents and children we can see that rearrangement of the relationship is possible. This can be done, however, only when we as parents give ourselves permission to look at ourselves and our needs and feelings first, so we can see what attitudes we have to change in order to adjust our relationships with our children. It is more difficult to change our behavior if it originates from our own unmet needs or feelings. Such a demand may make us want to blame the child for her problem. That would be less painful than recognizing and letting go of needs and feelings we have lived with all of our lives, or at least since becoming parents.

If you are a parent reading this book, you must continue to analyze relationships among all members of your family to understand how one of your children could infer that both nurturing and authoritative (protective) resources aren't available to her. After you have completed this rather exhaustive task (make sure you have support from another person before attempting it), plan how the family system can be changed and she can eventually—sporadically at first—seek support from other members of the family. The change in posture on your part must be consistent and won't even be rewarded for quite a while by your resistant anorexic daughter.

While the book will offer you insights, and a perspective on anorexia nervosa, what it cannot deliver is the tremendous amount of emotional energy your child's illness will require of you, if you are to defeat it. No doubt living with a victim of anorexia nervosa has already exhausted you, and the battle has yet to begin.

A few words to the victims of anorexia themselves: When one suffers from a psychological disorder, overcoming it means understanding its positive points—what you get out of having it. The most common "benefits" achieved by sufferers of anorexia nervosa as related to me over the past twenty-five years are:

—It makes me special.
—It proves I have more willpower to resist food than other girls.
—It's the only way I can say no to people (by refusing to gain weight).
—It's my assertiveness.
—I'm invisible without it.
—It's my friend.
—It gives me a sense of protection.

These are all "benefits" that eventually can be transferred to important people in your life to take the place of the "it." New ways are found to say "no" to others. Other forms of achievement are sought and developed. Ways of feeling visible are found. In general a reliable person or persons can replace all the "benefits" derived from having anorexia nervosa. If you have developed anorexia nervosa, however, you probably don't think much of my suggestions or feel optimistic about finding people whom you will be able to depend upon emotionally. Anorexia nervosa could well be called the "mistrusters' disease." Still, this becomes part of the recovery process: becoming vulnerable toward reliable persons, using them as guides and "mirrors" of your appearance and personality.

You are also, like so many other women, responding to the cultural message about reducing body fat to a minimum. This cultural message has come from women's service magazines, and has spread to Hollywood where we see actress after actress slim herself down to her wrinkled minimum. If the models are waif-thin, and the actresses follow suit, it must certainly seem that it is every girl and woman's obligation to be as slim as possible.

Men do not feel guilty if they fail the "pinch an inch" test, because a similar demand is not placed upon men. Perhaps we should examine our notions of femininity. Thinness has not always been the rule for women, but being alluring has. Alluring adornments on women can be seen on the walls of the pharaohs' tombs, so we know that this isn't a recent fad or cultural trend. Why then have women confused "allure" with being thin, and subsequently pursued this "correct" appearance? Obviously, to attract and sexually arouse men. Unaroused men do not function sexually. One might then view the origins of women's need to be alluring to the propagation of the species. This would mean that at its core femininity has two purposes: to attract men and nurture children. These are extremely politically incorrect statements to make in the late nineties. But if we understand that femininity *begins* with this goal, then we can understand how a commercialized society can transform this instinctive aspect of a girl or woman into the desire to have the "correct" body. The best way to capitalize on this need, then, is to make women hate their bodies when they are not dieting. Once women learn to hate their bodies they can be sold exercise products, gym and health club memberships, weight-loss programs, over-the-counter diet foods and drinks, athletic shoes, gym attire . . . the list is an endless merchandising blitz conceived by very creative advertising agencies and manufacturers. These societal changes, and the pressure on women to fit the image, target a very vulnerable segment of society: young girls just coming to grips with their femininity and eager to belong. These societal trends affecting women, family systems, and individual heredity have contributed in launching the onset of this psychological disorder. Regardless of the causes, changes in important relationships and psychotherapy, in some cases combined with medication, can help change the rather discouraging statistics on recovery from this extremely stubborn and tenacious personality-altering illness.

Anorexia nervosa has many "cousins," disorders that have similar personality characteristics: rigidity, perfectionism, inconsolability, detachment, mistrust, and repeated behaviors to reassure one's self and control anxiety. Most prominent among them are Obsessive-Compulsive disorders. There is much debate today about the causes of these illnesses in terms of psychological vs. hereditary/chemical reasons. Both of these illnesses, no doubt, contain elements of each, and for many victims it will mean both medication and psychotherapy. In the past eight years the progress in psychopharmacology—new medications for these illnesses—has taken a great leap forward.

With the increasing interest in treating anorexia nervosa by mental health professionals, doctors, and psychopharmacologists, we have more tools, understanding, and treatments than we have had in the past. We also have a clearer picture of the depth of the psychopathology, or mental illness, behind the victim's refusal to eat enough or to gain weight. We understand that there are issues relating to trust, identity, femininity, dependency, as well as family life, heredity, and cultural influences that must all be addressed with great energy and thoroughness in order to improve the rate of true recovery.

Much of the knowledge we need is now at hand. Our efforts to combat this insidious and tenacious disorder will continue. Hopefully, when you have finished reading this book you will no longer feel like a stranger to this disorder or to the victims who are suffering from it.

Steven Levenkron
May 1997

1

The Population and the Disease

Until recently, the victims of anorexia nervosa were almost exclusively upper-middle-class adolescent girls. In the past several years, however, because of more inclusive reporting and more accurate diagnosis—and to what is generally accepted by experts as an enormous increase in the incidence of the disease itself—the spectrum has been expanded to encompass all socioeconomic levels (though still 97 percent white). Age of onset has been broadened to include females from the ages of eleven to sixty (92 percent). The most common ages of onset remain between thirteen and twenty-two. Areas of the globe reporting this phenomenon include North America, Western Europe, and Australia. Most estimates place the disease's incidence at one out of every 250 adolescent girls. Unfortunately, government agencies and medical associations have little to offer us statistically. The estimated figures do not distinguish the duration of the illness for an individual patient, so the rate of increase in the total number of victims cannot be measured. If the recovery rate is low, we can be sure of rapidly escalating figures as new anorexics are added to the current chronically ill population.

Overcontrol of eating for weight reduction has recently been recognized as psychopathological behavior. It is this new behavior pattern, added to a list of long-established psychological disorders, that defines the syndrome that we call anorexia nervosa. Most of the following symptoms are familiar to us already:

1. *Phobias* concerning changes in bodily appearance are the illness's most outstanding feature.
2. *Obsessional thinking* about food and liquid intake constrict the mental activities of the anorexic.
3. *Obsessive-compulsive rituals* dominate much of the anorexic's day.
4. *Feelings of inferiority* about intelligence, personality, and appearance are common.
5. *Splitting,* or perceiving decisions and consequences in terms of polarities, is typical. The anorexic never sees choices as moderate, and fears making "mistakes." This results in an inability to make new decisions and leads to extremely rigid, repetitious behavior.
6. *Passive-aggressive behavior* often develops as parents and health professionals try to coerce the anorexic in what becomes a power struggle over eating and nutrition.
7. *Disinterest in sexuality* is often a personality characteristic of the anorexia nervosa syndrome and results from:
   (a) general immaturity and a need to see oneself as a child, to ward off feelings of parental abandonment
   (b) fear of intimacy, physical or emotional

    (c)   failure of father to romance daughter healthily, to offer affection and compliments

    (d)   In the case of maturity-onset anorexia nervosa, sexual energies are distracted by obsessional fears of weight gain and ritualistic behaviors—over-planning of meals, special ways of cutting foods.

8. *Delusional thinking develops,* especially with regard to body size and quantities of food ingested.

9. *Paranoid fears* of criticism from others are often experienced, especially with respect to being seen as "too fat."

10. *Depression* can be observed, particularly in the chronic anorexic.

11. *Anxiety* is alleviated only by weight loss and fasting.

12. *Denial* is used, along with delusional thinking, to keep the anorexic starving, exercising, and away from people as well as the food she needs. Basically, then, she denies her emaciated appearance while continuing to view others who are substantially heavier as thinner than herself.

The most outstanding personality traits seen in the entrenched or long-term anorexic include a conservative rigidity, outward compliance toward others alternating with temper-tantrum behavior, and repetitious or ritualistic patterns normal in the infant and toddler but not in the adolescent. Such infantile and childish behaviors suggest that the antecedents of this (usually) adolescent breakdown lie in early childhood. They emerge in adolescence under the pressure to separate from parents. Failure to accept a more adult-looking body (more separation from parents) leads the incipient anorexic to diet as a means of gaining control over fears of inadequacy, rejection by others, and unidentifiable fears.

Dieting triggers the breakdown of defenses that, up to this time, have kept the vulnerable personality functioning. All the symptoms of this regression to infantile traits blossom out of diet-related obsessions and activities the personality feels compelled to play out to protect herself from self-imposed threats. As with all obsessive-compulsive disorders, the obsessive ideas and the compulsive rituals increase in number and become more complex until almost all the anorexic's thoughts are involved with serving her disease. For example: An initial self-imposed rule stipulating a decrease in caloric intake on the part of the dieter evolves into more rules. These might include time of day each meal or snack is to be eaten, what food group it must come from, how hot it must be, what size and color plate it must be placed on, how many pieces it must be cut into, and how much time must be spent eating.

Anorexia nervosa has to be seen as a "stylistic" breakdown resulting from cultural pressure, since it amounts to a pathological exaggeration of society's message to women. That message has been with us as a pervasive problem for more than a decade and a half, and the incidence of anorexia nervosa has escalated dramatically during the last five years. A generation of young girls and women has been indoctrinated by the thin ethic. One has only to review magazine fashion advertisements and television commercials over the past fifteen years to observe the relentless thinning of models. Epidemiological studies will surely show a parallel between this development and the disorder of emaciation.

The disorder becomes a disease when psychopathology becomes physiopathology—that is, when problems of the mind create problems for the body.

Outwardly, most anorexics begin retreating from family and friends as their weight drops below nutritional and appearance norms. Social contact is shunned, as it may invite eating.

Anorexics don't like to be seen eating (or not eating), and eating becomes an extremely private activity. A sense of vulnerability, shame, and competition for thinness becomes attached to food. Meal planning becomes a major preoccupation throughout the day. It is not uncommon for the anorexic to start cooking for the entire family—to take control of all eating and food shopping in the household. Such control of the total home food environment represents the kind of overworking and overthinking that characterizes the illness. The anorexic manages everyone's eating agenda in order to guarantee control over her own.

Other areas of overcontrolling often involve time or timing of events in the day. This too reflects a fear of disorganized eating and the need to overorganize everything to avoid chaotic consumption of food. Behavior becomes riddled with devices to minimize and forestall eating. Rituals of cutting up food, eating only certain types of food (minimal in carbohydrates), eating in minute forkfuls or very slowly to prolong gratification of the tiny quantities—these are a few of the common "protections" against overeating used by the anorexic.

Fears that others will become skinnier than she is become a paranoid focus for the anorexic. She continually compares her body with the bodies of other girls and women and sees herself, delusionally, as heavier. She fears that others will reject her for being too heavy or, in later stages of the illness, that she will be neglected for not being "especially" thin. As dieting moves from the appropriate to the pathological, feelings about weight and eating evolve from elation with first weight loss into competitive desperation in the insatiable pursuit of thinness.

Disordered eating behavior falls into three categories.

1. *Intake limiting*. This kind of anorexia nervosa involves extremely low intake of calories (300–600 per day) and is often accompanied by low liquid intake. A full stomach is equated with obesity. In some cases, a full bladder is assessed in the same way. Sensations from the stomach such as gas, gurgling, fullness, and pain are experienced in a highly exaggerated manner. Fears of overeating as well as of abdominal distention become an added factor. The controls imposed on eating tend to be unrelenting in this form of the illness.

2. *Anorexia/bulimia*. This form of the eating disorder is characterized by alternating bouts of starving and overeating. These cycles vary in length. Some individuals starve all day, only to eat for hours at night. Preferred foods are usually high in sugar and carbohydrates. Also common is a cycle of one to several days of near fasting followed by a day of heavy eating. Rising and falling blood sugar levels of girls and women in this group create mood swings that contribute to general emotional chaos and feelings of incompetence. Untreated, this pattern may resolve itself in six months or continue indefinitely.

3. *Bulimarexia*. This term is now used to describe those who consume up to fifteen thousand calories in a day but vomit nearly all of it up to avoid weight gain. Individuals in this group vary from emaciated to normal. Although their eating practices differ from those of the first two groups, their thought processes and obsessions with eating and weight are similar. They become attached and addicted to the vomiting.

Within all three groups, there are individuals who further abuse their digestive systems by using laxatives, diuretics, enemas, and occasionally emetics in order to control weight.

I have seen diabetic anorexics attempt to manipulate insulin doses in the belief that this will help them to lose weight. They reduce or eliminate their use of insulin, putting themselves in severe danger of descending into a diabetic coma and, in any case, accelerating the deterioration of vision, teeth, and vital organs.

The anorexic is generally not the first-born child. I have found that in 80 percent of cases, the anorexic is the second or third child. She has a history of high achievement at school and is compliant and cooperative within the family. She is distinctly *not* in the spotlight at home—certainly not in any negative sense. She attracts little attention for her accomplishments and is careful to avoid criticism. Often someone else in the family is officially labeled the family problem—a sibling or parent with an identified chronic medical, mental, or emotional condition. Yet these dynamics may exist simply as the result of one family member's demanding the most attention. Typically, the potential anorexic is *not* this person.

The family of a child who develops anorexia nervosa can usually be characterized as "depleted" throughout most of the anorexic's childhood. This term refers to parents who for external reasons—that is, external demands on their energies—have outstripped their emotional resources. I also use the word to describe a parent or parents who suffer from chronic depression, anxiety, or other disabling feelings that prevent them from offering healthy nurturing. This is characterized by parents' inattention to and impatience with the child. Depletion of the parent(s) often results in an *implicit reversal of dependency* between parent and child. The parent's message to the child has been, "You have more strength than I." The child reacts by becoming the parent within the relationship. She assumes the role of assisting or supporting her parent(s) emotionally. She may become a high achiever, a pleaser of others. Such behavior is her contribution to raising family morale, or the morale of a depressed parent.

The parents of this child, then, come to welcome her strength and supportiveness, take it for granted, depend upon it. They give her too many decisions to make, too many options, and fail to see that she needs their emotional support. She learns to disregard reassurance—rarely provided when she's upset. Parent(s) further retreat from offering guidance to her. Thus, the anorexic is appreciated for what nurturing she offers other members of the family. She sees herself as being loved for *not* having needs of her own. This message teaches her that other people (such as her parents) can't make her feel safe. She must make herself safe! Rituals and overorganizing become her vanguard. She attempts frantically to assume responsibility for her own well-being. Since there is no one to fall back on emotionally, she must overthink and overwork in order to be perfect in all she does. It is as if she becomes answerable to an imagined parent, indeed an infantile parent who demands perfection or imposes rejection. This parent and the child live in symbiosis, stronger than any bond between real parent and child.

What looks good on the surface may, in fact, be quite the opposite. The child appears outgoing, cheery, and competent. This is her supportive behavior directed at what she sees as depleted parents. As she becomes ill, her anger toward her parents for being cast too early in life into the role of nurturer begins to emerge.

2

Evolution of the Illness

The individual pathological features just listed can be viewed as a constellation of separate symptoms. They interact to form an illness that develops momentum and dynamics of its own. The depression that an anorexic experiences, for instance, may be a reaction to her inability to stop the onslaught of obsessive ideas. She may feel hopeless about breaking free of compulsive behavior patterns. Her fear of socializing may grow out of a fear of having to eat with others.

PSYCHOLOGICAL ONSET

This occurs when an individual is no longer acting (or dieting) out of choice but out of a compulsion. Many adolescent girls have been put, or have put themselves, on diets. Since dieting involves a change in nutritional patterns as well as appearance (crucial to most adolescents), it is a serious step to take during a volatile period in human emotional development. Today's adolescent dieter is aiming to achieve a more acceptable appearance together with feelings of greater control over her eating behavior and weight. If she has healthy, trusting relationships with family and friends, she will be able to diet within a realistic set of norms. If she is a loner who does not form intimate relationships with others, she may be dieting from an unhealthy fear of disapproval or an abstract need to compete with others to win "thinnest" status. Either of these motivations can lead to the onset of anorexia nervosa.

Dieting is stressful behavior for most of us and could be labeled "obsessogenic" in nature. None of us diets casually; when we are dieting we think about it much of the time. When the dieter drifts away from socially accepted dieting norms, she is relinquishing lifelines to a healthy perspective. With the loss of such perspective, she is drawn toward obsessive isolation. As her thoughts become nearly all food/weight/exercise-related, she loosens her emotional connections to others. Obsessive thoughts inspire imaginary arenas in which to compete—for lowest weight, greatest weight loss, most intense exercise program. Once she becomes enmeshed in these arenas, she is lost to others as a recipient of guidance.

It is during this incipient period that guidance from key persons can prevent the development of acute illness. Once the imaginary arenas have been entered, and real social and familial areas abandoned, the momentum of the illness will build and the patient will have a clinical case of anorexia nervosa.

CLINICAL DIAGNOSIS

The criteria for clinical diagnosis include

- loss of 20 percent of body weight
- loss of the menstrual period
- thinning hair
- dry, flaking skin
- constipation
- lanugo—a downy growth of body hair
- lowered blood pressure—80/50 is not uncommon
- lowered body temperature—97°–95°F
- lowered chloride levels (if vomiting)
- lowered potassium levels (if vomiting)
- lowered pulse rate—60–39 bpm

These clinical conditions show how serious the illness has become. A patient presenting extreme clinical data is also undergoing extreme psychological disturbance. It is difficult to understand whether the data are an indication of how far the patient has damaged herself physically because of her emotional disturbance, or how severely her metabolic disturbances affect her mind. What we do know is that anorexic patients in severe metabolic distress present signs of severe emotional distress. Continuous medical supervision of a patient presenting these physiological manifestations of distress is necessary for her safety as well as for psychotherapeutic value. Management of the patient involves a mental health practitioner and a physician working as a team.

ACUTE STAGE

This stage is characterized by continuing weight loss and multiplying symptoms of nutritional deprivation. The patient is psychologically ''committed'' to anorexic thinking and behavior patterns. Her receptivity to guidance or counseling will be poor; intensive psychotherapy becomes imperative at this point. The patient may have been unnoticed or treated ineffectively up to this time.

Psychologically, the patient has developed food- and weight-related rituals (these include limiting food intake and exercising beyond reason—biking, running, doing hundreds of push-ups, sit-ups, and deep knee-bends, clearly to excess relative to her physical and nutritional states). She is fearful of becoming obese or changing any eating patterns, and she is delusional about her body. She views herself as heavier than those around her. She often sees the appearance of others accurately but distorts her own appearance by contrast: "Yes, she's really thin, but I'm much heavier than she is." (This is a typical delusional contrast made by an emaciated anorexic patient.)

During this acute stage, she is consolidating recently formed eating and drinking patterns that tend to allow only minimal consumption. Timing and privacy become important with regard to eating. It is very painful if not intolerable for the anorexic to have her parents present while she is eating. She will eat at another time, or in the solitude of her room. At this stage a power struggle in defense of the illness begins.

The formerly compliant personality suddenly becomes defiant and secretive—but only in the area of weight control. She readily dismisses others' perceptions of her appearance and nutritional needs. She is socially inactive and engaged in battles at home over her eating (and, in many cases, her excessive exercising). Her parents describe her as rigid and tyrannical. They are often intimidated by her aggressiveness as well as by the evidence of her illness. The anorexic frequently believes she's unlikable, homely, unintelligent, and so on, and hopes that by achieving the "perfect" weight she will ward off those feelings.

The anorexic develops a special pattern of *simplifying*, of displacing all fears and concerns onto the area of weight. Solutions are likewise dependent on losing weight. The obsessive system includes a system of rewards and punishments: if she is "good," she may eat more today; if she is unproductive, she will be prohibited from eating. The allowable amounts to be eaten as rewards tend to fall below minimal. Distortion is applied to quantities eaten. The anorexic may fast for a day, then eat a 200-calorie dinner and become frightened that she has eaten too much. It is not unusual for a patient to state (as an indication of improvement), "I ate a hot fudge sundae today," meaning that little else has been consumed.

If the patient makes this kind of statement after a therapeutic alliance has been formed, she is not consciously being deceptive; she is torn between pleasing the therapist she is learning to trust, and the voice in her head to which she has become answerable. She tries to please them both, still owing primary loyalty to the "imaginary mother" who demands perfection. It is the shifting of this primary loyalty from the "imaginary mother" to the therapist that is the core of therapeutic change. The therapist's role in establishing the therapeutic alliance is described in Chapter 3 and amplified in Chapters 4 through 8.

THE ENTRENCHED STAGE

This stage, which could also be called the chronic stage, refers to the length of time an individual has been living an anorexic existence. Long-term anorexics (five to forty years) are much harder to treat because (1) the patterns of the illness have become intrinsic to their personalities; (2) their need for intimate contact with others has diminished; (3) their sense of hopelessness about themselves has become accepted; and (4) their cynicism about psychotherapists and other professionals who failed them (and sometimes mistreated them) prevents them from wanting to "start again."

In most instances, the chronic anorexic has tailored her environment to her illness, and those around her have resigned themselves to it. She may control the schedule and content of meals. She may even do the family food shopping and arrange the refrigerator and pantry. This kind of patient needs a milieu that will support change—whether a hospital or other residential treatment center.

THE CRISIS OF RECOVERY

Anorexia nervosa can be characterized as an attachment to a sadistic, imaginary mother, invented to fill a nurturing (and often a power) vacuum. Recovery is tantamount to separation from that parent. The tenaciousness with which an anorexic clings to her symptoms represents a major challenge to the energies of the therapist. It becomes the therapist's task to create this separation and to help the patient deal with the terror that accompanies it. The therapist, in a sense, is in competition with the (imaginary mother) illness. The therapist must instill in the patient not only a will to recover but a *reason* to recover. The therapeutic relationship must offer the patient as much security as the illness does.

The patient has been using *magical thinking* to feel safe. Ultimately, she becomes a slave to that magical thinking. Most young children use magical thinking to calm their anxieties about the unknown, but as the real world offers them more safety, they begin to give up the imaginary world. The anorexic, however, has returned to magical thinking, creating individual superstition-spawned rituals, and she shuns the real world. Essentially, this is because she has not received the kind of emotional nurturing that would allow her to trust herself to cope with the more adult tasks ahead—tasks that involve adolescent social and sexual demands, and school and career decisions that will separate her from her parents.

The therapist must make reality more attractive to the anorexic and give her confidence that she will have sufficient power over herself, her impulses, and her life. She views herself in dichotomous terms: either she will be in charge of everything (simplified into eating and weight), or she will be powerless (fat). The patient must be taught to trust the therapist first, so that she may then learn to trust herself. Developing trust in another person, at the expense of obsessive ideas, usually precipitates a crisis that ends in recovery.

Recovery begins with heightened anxiety that cannot be moderated by the patient's obsessive defense system. (Until now, by focusing on weight loss, she has managed to suppress anxieties over other issues and worries.) If the trust-based anxiety is strong enough to change eating behavior, the crisis of recovery has begun. Eating will increase unevenly and the patient will be frightened that her weight gains demonstrate loss of control. She will also be afraid of losing her uniqueness and of becoming undeserving of attention. At this point, the therapist must help the patient understand that she will retrieve—even enhance—the richness and complexity of her personality.

Recovery takes several paths. With the "new" anorexic who has been ill for less than a year, recovery is characterized by a constant weight gain of two to three pounds a week, until the patient is at a low but acceptable weight. Patients whose weight was normal when they began dieting (85 percent do not have overweight problems) usually stop gaining weight and remain several pounds below the preanorexic weight. Psychologically, they will be frightened and preoccupied with the dreaded prospect of overeating and becoming overweight for months after having reached safe weight levels. These fears and obsessions will gradually subside in from six weeks to eighteen months.

Setbacks during recovery are common, especially with the chronic anorexic. Changes in the family, school pressures, discharge from a hospital, arguments with important people in the patient's life—all may affect her eating behavior. If the patient is hospitalized, a compliment by a physician or nurse, such as "You're looking better" is perceived as "You're looking fatter." During the weight-recovery period, or "refeeding," many such incidents may interfere with the steady gaining of weight.

CONSOLIDATION OF RECOVERY

One of the major fears of the chronic and even the short-term anorexic is that the entire world wants only to "fatten her up." Her weight loss and her eating behavior are symptoms. They are truly dazzling and terrifying symptoms to family and medical community alike, but they are only the symptoms of underlying emotional difficulties. This is something that must be stated and restated to the recovering anorexic lest she return to her rituals to bring about relief from unresolved fears.

Achieving a true recovery from anorexia nervosa means that the patient understands and appreciates her complexity, and relinquishes the need to retreat to obsessive simplification of emotional conflict. The patient must again be able to form satisfactory intimate relationships with peers and to turn to others for help and security. Recovery also means developing flexibility and decision-making skills. Many of these desirable outcomes of successful psychotherapy for the anorexic can be traced back to the central issue, trusting oneself. If she can be taught to trust herself, she will be able to trust herself in relationships with others and to trust her ability not to be hurt. She can trust her decision making and her ability to live with decisions made. Developing a sense of trust where none has existed means reconstructing a developmental building block formed defectively in the early years of childhood. This can take from two to five years. It is impossible to predict with any one patient how long a course of therapy will take, but it is useful to have some approximate limits.

3

Toward a Nurturant-Authoritative Psychotherapy

Traditional psychotherapeutic training presumes a neutral attitude on the part of the therapist. That neutrality has been defended as protection for the patient from "nonobjective" behavior by the therapist. The neutral position or posture also encourages patient growth, elicits patient rage, and finally encourages the patient to see that it is the patient's nonobjective behavior that must be corrected. With the correction of this behavior comes maturity, rationality, and mental health. If the therapist "behaves" in a particular manner toward the patient, the therapist is then labeled a manipulator. The assumption is that the therapist is manipulating for personal needs and out of lack of respect for the patient's ability to arrive at the proper answers autonomously. It would seem that the closer the therapist comes to being "nobody," the better the quality of the therapy.

There are other self-serving and self-protecting aspects

attached to what might be termed passive-therapist behavior. This posture limits the responsibility of the therapist and places "blame" on the patient for thoughts and ideas that the patient experiences. No one can accuse the passive therapist of sadistic, aggressive, seductive, or hostile behaviors. These become the products of the patient's imagination, or "transference." The passive posture relieves the therapist of responsibility for taking the initiative or using creative energy while doing therapy. Should the patient love or hate the therapist, that is interpreted as the patient's transference of feelings about parental figures onto the therapist. Thus, the therapist is immune from evaluation by the patient.

A nurturant-authoritative psychotherapy demands more initiative, more tactical decision making, and more varied, deliberate behavior on the part of the therapist than does traditional therapy. Juxtaposed with traditional psychotherapy, the nurturant-authoritative therapist's first task is to regress the patient—to help the patient become younger and less mature within the therapeutic relationship.

My experience is that nurturant-authoritative (NA) psychotherapy helps the patient with anorexia nervosa learn to accept and receive emotional support. The therapist takes the explicit role of a helping person who has ways of guiding the patient out of her lonely and pathological state. The therapist must be willing to provide supportive talk, especially in the beginning phases of therapy. Interminable silences are destructive to the anorexic patient.

Interventions—the term used to describe the verbal responses of the therapist to the patient—assume a different meaning in NA therapy. Many traditional psychoanalytic responses like "What do *you* think about that?" or "You'll know when you're ready" are *abandoning interventions* in NA therapy. These are responses that leave the floundering anorexic patient more convinced than ever that she is on her own and that there is no help for her. They tend to reflect her parents' passive and dependent behavior toward her.

Following are some of the passive-dependent remarks parents make to anorexic children who are too young to use the initiative that is prematurely thrust upon them.

"You've always been smarter than me."

"You're too hard to understand."

"You've always been able to figure things out for yourself best."

"How can I help you?"

"Help me to help you."

A young person who hears this needs an authority figure, and the NA therapist's task is to become established as a confident—therefore attractive—person who has something to offer. The patient has often been rewarded for not needing dependence, for not needing assistance, for not needing guidance, for *not needing*. Needing equals failing. The job of the therapist is to help the patient be able to need.

It is not hard to see how *needing to eat* has become connected in this patient's mind with failing. The NA therapist, then, has to help the patient feel need for the assistance of another person and accept the feeling of dependence, to develop dependency in a person who shuns it. The therapist must develop a care-taking relationship with someone who views relationships as always competitive. The patient must see the therapist as nurturer offering care, as authority figure offering guidance. The therapist must help the patient feel safe when *she* isn't controlling the nurturing. This patient has always felt safest when "offering." She feels most helpless when "receiving" or waiting to receive.

Another facet of NA therapy is its explicitness about the process of therapy. Passive behavior on the part of the therapist explains nothing about the therapy process to the patient, making it part of the patient's therapeutic task to decipher the therapy process. This repeats what has happened at home, where the child or woman has received many implicit messages and inferred that she is responsible for those around her. If nobody explains the process of therapy to her, she is again free to infer that she is uncared for, unnurtured.

INTERVENTIONS OF INTERPRETATION

Therapists have many responsibilities toward their patients. They provide information, explain the therapeutic process, and interpret the patient's thoughts, dreams, and behavior—especially behavior within the therapeutic meetings. This last task is an important part of the NA therapist's role. The therapist must be able to demonstrate that he or she *understands* the patient, accomplishing this by interpreting the unspoken, the gesture, even the silence. During initial meetings, the therapist should stay with those generalizations about anorexia that convince the patient that he or she understands the illness. This will relieve the patient's fears of being misunderstood as well as demonstrate that her therapist has taken the trouble to study her particular problem.

Such behavior by a therapist, in traditional psychotherapy parlance, would be criticized as "premature interpretation." In NA therapy, it serves as a support tool for developing trust and also demystifying the patient's illness to her. In the context of eating disorder therapy, this might be termed "spoonfeeding." Since this type of patient has not been able to accept emotional spoonfeeding in the past, this is experienced by her as verbal nurturing. The therapist's behavior must reflect supportiveness, expertise, the ability to guide and structure, sensitivity to her obsessive traps, and confidence in the ability to help her. This behavior must balance nurturing and offering care with authoritativeness and an ability to structure the therapeutic relationship sympathetically.

The nurturant/authoritative balance must be maintained. If the therapist were only to nurture, the patient would soon become angry, contemptuous, and, finally, manipulative and tyrannical. Open-ended nurturing would be experienced by the patient as weak—nice but impotent. This would reinforce the patient's background, and the therapist would be seen as another passive-dependent person, incapable of offering her the kind of strength she would find both safe and attractive.

If the therapist, on the other hand, were to behave authoritatively without establishing a bond through nurturing, the patient might learn to fear the therapist and, in some cases, comply with demands for weight gain. In many behavior-modification programs, authoritativeness is the main tool. This produces cosmetic progress as it drives the patient back to her previous posture of being a "good little girl." In a hospital setting, the authoritative approach can become an authoritarian approach. When this is used, the patient gains weight to escape the clutches of her captors. Once free of their control, she often loses the weight she gained in fearful compliance with their demands. In out-patient therapy, the authoritative therapist merely turns off the patient and produces passive-withdrawn behavior. There is no progress, but there is a great deal of deception on the part of the patient.

Obviously, either posture—by itself—becomes a simplified extreme, one that would put the therapist in the same trap as the patient, who can see issues only in polarities. As the therapist struggles to maintain a balance, the patient learns from this behavior that issues are complex, and solutions often must be the result of negotiated moderation—the antithesis of obsessive thinking.

The role of the therapist, then, is to reconcile and balance two postures that are typically seen as antithetical. As a result, he or she will help his patient feel protected and released from obsessive chaos.

4

Lonnie

Lonnie G., an attractive sixteen-year-old girl, five feet seven inches tall, was admitted to the hospital weighing 82 pounds. She expressed fears about being in the hospital but because of her fright, confusion, and disorientation she appeared resigned to being hospitalized. She had been identified as anorexic by her family physician eight months earlier. Her weight dropped from 125 to 105. At 105 she stopped menstruating but persisted in limiting her caloric intake to 400 per day. Despite admonitions from her parents, friends, and physician, she continued losing weight. Her mother described Lonnie as having become increasingly withdrawn as her weight dropped. In issues not related to eating and exercising (she did two hours of calisthenics a day), Lonnie was passive and glum. Mrs. G. described her daughter as a "try-hard kid": "Whatever it is, she gives it her all." Mrs. G. also mentioned that

Lonnie's two older brothers were high achievers, both in college.

Lonnie had been seeing a psychiatrist for six months. In addition to psychotherapy, the psychiatrist had placed Lonnie on Thorazine, an antipsychotic drug, and Elavil, an antidepressant. The psychiatrist reasoned that these would be an aid to psychotherapy, since the first drug would calm Lonnie's fears about gaining weight, and the Elavil had been suggested by a colleague of his for its presumed antianorectic side effects.

The psychiatrist had asked Lonnie about school, friends, getting along with family members, wishes, fears, hopes she had—to no avail. He felt it was not helpful to talk about weight or eating since he did not want to be seen in the same role as her mother or father.

Mrs. G. explained that her daughter had become more retiring when she entered high school in the ninth grade. "There was never any cause for worry about that girl. I'm shocked at what's happened to her in the last year. We're a close family, not 'huggy-kissy,' but we all know that we care about each other. I'm sure Lonnie's brothers pushed her about a bit when they were all younger, but nothing beyond normal." Mr. G. described himself as a quiet man. "I don't make a lot of noise, but I do what is required. My wife's a bit on the nervous side but not about Lonnie, not until all this."

Lonnie enters the Adolescent Medicine office for her first session and docilely sits down. I stare at what appears to be a blank face, then say to her, "Are you scared?"

She nods. I move my chair within three feet of hers and ask her if she is frightened of being in the hospital.

She looks up at me. "Yes."

"Are you scared of gaining weight?"

She is beginning to look more frightened. "Yes."

To indicate to her that I understand what she is going through, I ask her if she is scared all the time.

She responds with a surprised and emphatic "Yes!"

I say, "I can help you not to be scared. I'm going to be in charge of you and you'll be safe." I watch her confused expression. She notices me watching. I nod. "Yes, I think you're going to need a lot of help. Help with understanding your feelings about your appearance, about your chances for success with other people, career, growing up—oh, yes, you'll need a lot of help. Now tell me, *how* scary is eating to you?"

She starts to cry. "I haven't eaten in four days and I can't anymore."

I hold a tissue up to her nose. "Blow," I instruct her. She looks surprised.

"Go ahead, blow." She blows her nose.

"When was the last time someone wiped your nose?" She laughs.

Initial clinical interviews usually serve two purposes: they enable the clinician to make an appraisal, evaluation, or diagnosis of the patient's condition; and if the patient is seeking psychotherapeutic treatment from the interviewing clinician, then the first interview sets the tone and structure for the developing therapeutic relationship. Unfortunately, too much emphasis is placed on the observations made by the clinician and too little on his or her behavior toward the patient. The clinician's or therapist's behavior affects the patient's behavior and may alter the diagnosis. It certainly affects the style of the therapeutic relationship that is taking shape.

The therapist's behavior is expected to be friendly in the passive sense, and inquiring. This is no doubt the safest behavior for the general clinical interview. When an anorexic patient is referred for therapy, however, she comes to the meeting resisting and resenting the fact of needing therapy, and more suspicious of the therapist than the average person who is actively seeking psychotherapy. She sees others as having failed her, but more importantly she sees herself as a failure in establishing relationships. She has little hope and even less energy for the establishment of the therapeutic relationship. She appears "flat," depressed, withdrawn, and impoverished in her ability to answer questions in an open, extended manner.

This last feature, the inability to answer questions in an extended manner, is what often sabotages the building of a helpful therapeutic relationship. The therapist has been trained to ask questions and to be able to wait out the patient, to allow extraordinary time for her to answer. So the patient feels like a failure for not being able to provide "better" answers for the therapist, and she interprets the silences as the therapist's disinterest in her. She often feels more hopeless and "unhelped" after such an interview than before it.

Since Lonnie is emaciated at the time of her initial interview, the following physical, medical, and social conditions exist:

- Lonnie has been obsessed by thoughts of eating, starving, controlling her weight, and exercising.
- She has lost contact with most of her friends.
- Her relationship with her parents is distant. She may seem to cling to them but can't talk to them or experience security in the clinging.
- Lonnie has difficulty sleeping, because of her low weight.

- Sitting and lying down are uncomfortable, as she has no fat tissue for padding.
- She is always cold, as her body temperature is below normal.
- In short, Lonnie comes to her first therapy session as a frightened, cold, lonely, starved, and physically tortured, exhausted person—not unlike an actual concentration camp inmate.

It is my task to indicate to Lonnie that I can understand and identify the nature of her imprisonment. That Lonnie has imprisoned herself makes no difference at this point. She has the personality makeup of one who is imprisoned by others. She has also learned that no one has been able to offer her confident understanding. This confident, understanding posture can mitigate Lonnie's feelings that her illness is stronger than anyone's ability to rescue her.

As her therapist I, in effect, announce that I intend to rid Lonnie of this illness. My holding a tissue to her nose is a way of offering her physical (parental) care. The parental nature of the physical care expressed helps Lonnie to become younger, regressed, within the therapeutic relationship. The NA therapist has to be the kind of individual who is comfortable as both a nurturer and an authoritative person. He or she may have to overcome previous psychoanalytic taboos that characterize such behavior as seductive, intrusive, "acting out," and manipulative. It is just this quality of active behavior that the professionally aware NA therapist uses to develop a regressive relationship with the patient. Such a relationship will help the patient view the therapist as more potent than the obsessive thinking to which she has surrendered.

"How can you help me when I can't even eat?"

"At our next meeting I will bring breakfast and help you eat it."

"I'll be too scared to eat it."

"Yes, you'll be scared, but you'll be able to eat, even though it will frighten you. I will help you deal with the fear so you can eat. Being frightened doesn't mean you can't do it. It does mean you need someone who can make you feel safe enough to tolerate breaking your own restrictions on eating."

"But I'll be scared after."

"We'll talk afterward until you're not frightened about having eaten the meal."

"But what if I'm scared later in the day?"

"You'll call me and I'll calm you down."

Lonnie still looks worried, but the severity of her anxiety has clearly been tempered by the stable posture of the therapist.

I bring breakfast for Lonnie into the office for our second session. Opening the container that holds two scrambled eggs and toast, I announce the menu and place a container of milk on the desk. Lonnie looks at the food. She appears bewildered. Blank spaces and silences invite obsessing at moments when decision making is required. I hand her a knife and a fork.

"Now just begin to eat," I say in an upbeat manner, as if I were teaching a child how to swim who had never been in deep water before. Nervously she pulls herself toward the desk and woodenly places forkfuls of egg and bites of toast into her mouth.

"Try not to eat too fast and have some milk."

She reaches for the milk, opens the familiar school-lunchroom-sized container, places the straw in it, and begins drinking. Her motions are automatonlike, as if she doesn't want to know that she is eating. She is anesthetized to what is happening. I keep talking, reassuring her that she will not have to be alone with these fears and at the same time making it clear that she has to keep eating. At this point, I am coaching her eating in much the same way an athletic coach gets a player through a new task—reassuring, demanding, and cheering her on. She finishes the meal at a rapid pace and looks relieved when the eating is over.

"Now let's talk about how frightened you feel about having eaten this meal."

"I feel very frightened." She is trying to control the fear in her voice.

"You're frightened because you think you're going to gain weight from what you've just eaten." It is not a question, simply a recognition of what she is ashamed to say aloud.

She nods. I go into a lengthy explanation about digestion, absorption of food by the intestines, and elimination. "Only a small portion of what you ate will be absorbed by your body, and even that is far below what is needed to maintain your present weight. I will help you to get to the point where you *are* eating enough to gain weight. We want to overcome your fears connected with those words and those ideas. And this is probably a good time to talk about how weight will come on—specifically where it will appear, and in what order."

"But I know I'll gain it in my stomach first. After I eat, my stomach sticks out so much! Look at it!" She stands up, looks around as if she were searching for a place to run. The mounting panic is clearly visible.

"I would like to tell you what *I* see." I point to her abdomen. "Your stomach is distended because you have just filled it up. But the first place you put on weight is not your abdomen. For the first hour after you eat, while food is being digested, the upper part of your abdomen protrudes. Then as food passes through your intestines, the lower part of the abdomen protrudes. Ordinarily, this is not so obvious. The reason you seem to 'stick out' so much is that you're contrasting what you see now with a totally empty digestive system. You have absolutely no fat tissue on your hips. So, in essence, the thinner you get the more you "stick out" when you eat, especially when that eating is irregular and you're going directly from empty to full."

Anorexics need to believe that they are perpetually on the borderline of weighing too much. They utilize this fear of overweight to maintain their obsessive self-discipline. It becomes important for the therapist to examine the patient's visual perceptions of herself and then reinterpret them for her. In effect, the therapist is saying, "You are confused about your appearance; I am more objective. You may utilize my objectivity to calm yourself." The explanation made to this patient is repeated after each meal she has with the therapist, and may be used by a nurse if one is available to eat with her.

The therapist then needs to explain where weight will appear. There is a temptation to be intimidated by the anorexic's fears and to refrain from discussion of actual weight gain. This would be an error and would be interpreted by the patient as the therapist's fear of her really gaining weight.

"Weight gain does *not* begin in your stomach. It begins in your lower buttocks, then your upper buttocks, then thighs, calves, hips, rib cage, arms, and breasts. Nature takes care to make sure you'll have enough muscle to stand and walk, so it develops the most important muscles first. If you want to determine whether or not you are gaining weight, see if your coccyx is still protruding." Pointing to her coccyx (a small bone at the base of the spinal column), I say, "Go ahead, Lonnie, touch that protruding bone." She touches her coccyx. "Do you notice that it hurts when you sit on a hard surface or slide against the back of a chair?"

She nods.

"Well, nature didn't mean for that bone to stick out, and when it does, it means you're too thin. So as you increase your eating, check to see if your coccyx is receding. It should recede as you begin to build up your upper buttocks. You will also notice that you can sit more comfortably and walk more steadily. *Never* try to decide about your weight from looking at your stomach. That's one of the last places you will put on weight, though it *is* the first part of your body to *look* larger."

Lonnie is both reassured and shaken by this information. She looks at her arms. They are severely emaciated and the excess skin lies in folds at the shoulder and elbow joints. She grabs at the skin folds in a pinching motion. "What about this? Look at this fat!"

"No, that isn't fat. It's the absence of fat." I am combating her distortion with repetitious reality. "Your body has reduced beyond your skin's ability to shrink. Now you have excess skin with not enough underneath it. You have become too thin for your own skin, so it hangs in folds like a garment that is too large on you. You see, Lonnie, you are interpreting the absence of fat as fat. It's shriveled skin that you're confusing with fat."

Lonnie thinks over the explanation about her shriveled skin. "It looks like fat. It must be fat." Again she is escalating toward that self-induced panic.

"No, it's skin." I repeat this in a very matter-of-fact tone.

Emphasizing the patient's confusion to her, in the initial phase of treatment, helps to establish the therapist as a knowledgeable person to be depended upon. The therapist doesn't become angry or impatient, as her family has. Instead, the therapist will continue to explore distortion and examine in detail the patient's feelings about her body. The therapist will clarify the patient's misperceptions repeatedly. These clarifications, offered sympathetically, will serve as an emotional reservoir of thinking to combat her obsessive ideas. The information that the therapist offers the patient is still only a tool, however. The therapist must be seen as a dependable person so that the therapeutic relationship will provide the leverage required to move the patient out of her lonely, obsessive trap.

"Lonnie, since you're frightened about what you look like, why don't you tell me what you're afraid others will see when they look at you?"

"They'll see how fat I am and they'll think I have no control."

"Do you think about this when you're in school?"

She wants to put a determined expression on her face, but her eyes will only stare blankly as her mouth tightens. The expression changes to resignation, the voice to despair. "I think people are thinking about how fat I am everywhere I go. When I walk down the street,

I'm sure everyone around me is thinking about how fat I am."

"Even just before you came into the hospital? Even when your weight was this low?"

She nods.

"It seems that you have only one problem."

She looks puzzled. I continue. "Your only problem is that you look too fat and the only solution to your only problem is to starve. It sounds pretty simple to me. I think you have really simplified your life. You don't have to worry about what people think of your intelligence, your character, whether you're interesting or dull, whether you're talented or not, likable or not. All you have to worry about is whether you're fat or not. In a way, it sounds like a good deal."

Lonnie is crying quietly.

"Why are you crying?"

"But sometimes I do think about all those things you said. When I do, it's terrible. I think everyone thinks I'm dull, dumb, boring, weak, and just nothing." She cries more intensely.

"When you're this upset about the rest of your problems, do you—right now—feel as upset about food and eating?"

She shakes her head. "But I know I will in an hour."

"Let's stay with these ideas about feeling dull, dumb, weak, and all the other things you just mentioned."

"What about them?"

"Are these ideas you've had about yourself for a long time?"

"Always."

"If you've had these ideas about yourself, it makes a

lot of sense to me that you would *prefer* to be frightened around the issue of your weight.''

She is annoyed. ''I don't *prefer* to be frightened about anything. I'm sick and tired of being frightened all the time. I'm frightened when I wake up, all day, and when I go to sleep. I hardly sleep, and when I'm dreaming it's usually about food, eating, and gaining too much weight. How could anybody *prefer* to live like I do?''

''I'm not suggesting that you want to be unhappy. But if you are unhappy, it still seems curious that most of the time you are only aware of your unhappiness over eating and weight.''

''I have no time to be aware of other things. I always have to think food, eating, overweight. If I don't, I'll get too fat!''

At this point, Lonnie has slipped back into believing that the only danger confronting her is the anorexic obsession. I now must shift from interpreting content to an NA regressing posture.

''You won't get too fat. We will both redefine your appearance until you develop an accurate perspective. You won't have to become too fat in order to avoid being too thin.''

Lonnie has been anorexic for nine months. While at this point she would not qualify as an ''early identification'' (first two months), therapy needs to be aimed at moving her out of the seriously low weight range as soon as possible. With chronic or entrenched anorexics (two years and more), the investment in the symptoms has come to have a profound influence upon the personality, which compounds the problems of treatment.

It is more difficult for the chronic patient to learn to trust yet another therapist who may fail her as the others have. She may have become depressed and lost hope or the active desire to be rid of the illness. She may have trained members of her family to accept the illness. And she may have narrowed her life to a schedule revolving around eating and exercising rituals. In this case, she has become a well-adjusted anorexic. The long-term nature of her rigidity and her acceptance of the loneliness inherent in the illness make her less desirous of (or even capable of) developing a therapeutic relationship. Bringing Lonnie out of the seriously low weight range means precipitating a crisis of recovery (see Chapter Two). Merely to coerce her out of the low weight range would be to create a "cosmetic cure." This results from the patient's desire to be rid of the coercing therapist (or coercing therapeutic environment). She will affect compliance, but most often she will lose the weight again, once free of her coercers.

The therapeutic goal for Lonnie is to guide her out of the acute stage while she is in an emotional alliance with her therapist, whom she views as a friend, not a persecutor. This will cause Lonnie severe agitation, since she will not detach herself from her weight-gaining behavior but will identify herself as a person who is gaining weight and truly relinquishing her former source of safety—rigid weight control. The severity of the conflict engendered by this shift means that she needs highly supportive behavior from me. During this crisis of recovery, she is not able to understand her motives or to interpret her feelings. She remains continually in need of emotional support. I, as her therapist, also continually demand that she gain weight. Little intellectual, cognitive, or analytical work is done during this period.

Lonnie's crisis of recovery peaks between eight to ten weeks. She becomes more delusional about her appearance; she sees herself as becoming obese. I must focus, repeatedly and patiently, on reality testing with regard to her weight. Confident reassurances are offered to meet the litany of fears that she expresses. After the eight to ten weeks have elapsed, Lonnie's agitation subsides enough to deal with such issues as her relationships with various members of her family (the source of feelings of inferiority) and her desire to avoid close relationships with peers. These problems are common to most anorexics.

The major themes that may be attempted during the crisis of recovery are mistrust of self, and seeing alternatives in polarities. For example: "Why do you have to be too fat if you aren't too thin? . . . Why are achievements disastrous if they aren't perfect?"

5

Lonnie—Consolidating the Recovery Alliance

The crisis of recovery is stressful to the patient, and it can threaten the alliance between patient and therapist. Lonnie's weight drops three pounds during her first week in the hospital. She can eat only with me. It is necessary to place Lonnie on total parenteral (intravenous) nutrition. Specifically, a small-bore catheter is inserted surgically into her jugular system from a point on her chest near her right shoulder. The tube is threaded from a smaller vein into the superior vena cava, several inches above the heart. The fluids that move through this catheter meet all of Lonnie's nutritional needs. An electric infusion pump controls the flow of liquids. The flow is increased gradually over several days to a maximum of 160 cubic centimeters an hour, or two thousand calories per day.

Lonnie is frightened by this device, which, for the first several days, increases her weight by a pound a day. Lonnie wants me to rescue her from the hyperalimentation apparatus and its weight-contributing effects. But I must help her to tolerate the process—and keep her eating.

At this time, the meals with Lonnie have a new element.

Lonnie begins to eat a turkey sandwich. She hears the gurgling sound of the infusion pump, and pauses.

"It's hard for me to eat." She tightens her jaw.

"When you hear the sound of the pump, I guess it makes you feel as if food and weight were coming at you from all directions."

She looks surprised at my observation. "How did you know that? That's exactly how I feel!"

"It's very quiet in here. The only sounds are your eating and the machine pumping. You wince every time it starts."

She becomes agitated. "Can't you turn it off? I can't eat with it on. I don't need it anymore. I'm gaining too much weight! Look at me!"

"No. It shouldn't be turned off. It's protecting you. I know it's scary but the pump is under control, sensible control. As you eat more, we turn it down to make up for the number of calories you're eating. You *are* gaining weight, at a reasonable rate. I don't see any change in your appearance yet. I'll tell you when I do. Do you see any change?"

"My stomach looks worse than ever! I just feel fatter everywhere!" Frantically, she puts down the sandwich and points to her stomach, arms, and legs.

"Maybe when you say that you *feel* fatter, what you mean is you are scared."

"Scared about being fat!"

"No. I think that 'fat' and 'scared' mean the same to

you. The problem with using 'fat' to mean 'scared' is that we never find out what the *real* fears are, only the fake ones."

"I'm *really* afraid of being fat!"

"What would happen to you if you got fat?"

Her voice gets panicky. "Oh, I knew it! I'm going to be fat! You just said it!"

"No. I asked you what *would* happen if you got fat. What are you afraid of? I'm trying to understand what the concept of being fat means to you beyond an unattractive appearance. No one wants to become unattractive, but you threaten yourself continually with an unrealistic danger. Your reaction to this unlikely danger has taken over most of your thinking. So we must find out what ideas, fears, and consequences are attached to this 'fat.' "

"That would be so terrible!"

"Would people stop liking you? Would you lose friends? Would your parents forget about you? Would people think you were stupid?"

"Yes, all of that!"

"If I gained five or ten pounds, Lonnie, would you not want to talk to me?"

"No." She becomes calmer. "Of course not."

"What if I gained it all in my stomach?"

"No!" She is indignant. "That wouldn't matter to me."

"Do you think other people who know me might care about me less?"

"No. Of course not." She looks puzzled.

"You seem surprised that I asked you these questions, Lonnie."

"Well, it's different for you. You're already somebody. You have a job and a family." Becoming tearful, she stares at the floor in front of her. "I'm nobody, nothing special. I've never been special in any way . . . to anyone. Having *this* is probably the most special thing I've ever done. I didn't do this to be special, but I'm beginning to feel like if I don't have this illness or disease, or whatever it is, then I'm going to be forgotten again. You won't need to see me when I look like everyone else."

"Do you believe that the only way you can become special is to be sick?"

"Well, up to now, that's the only way anybody's ever noticed me."

"Lonnie, I'm afraid just gaining weight alone won't do."

"What do you mean?"

"Our working relationship continues until you don't need help with understanding your moods and feelings any more, and I would guess that's a long way down the road."

"How long?"

"Oh, I'm afraid you're going to be stuck with talking to me for a couple of years."

"Are you sure?"

"Promise."

Lonnie looks relieved.

"I'm going to ask you to do a lot of things that are difficult to do."

"Like gaining weight?"

"Yes, that's the first issue to get out of the way. What we will have to reestablish, often, is that weight is *not* the real issue. It feels like the real issue but it is a catch-all for the varied and complex things that bother you. Now we will try to identify the kinds of ideas and feelings you have about yourself that trouble you. We will also have to talk about interactions between you and each member of your family, so we can understand how these ideas and feelings of yours developed.''

The anorexic patient does not come to therapy with the sophistication of most people entering psychoanalysis. She often comes involuntarily and is unfamiliar with the process of psychotherapy. The therapist has to help her enter into this special relationship. This involves teaching her how to be an active participant in her own therapy. With many adolescents, a basic explanation of psychotherapy is useful. In many cases, the patient comes from a family that regards psychotherapy as an alien idea. Her parents may even feel hostile toward having their daughter in therapy. They suddenly find themselves referred to professionals about whom they may have all sorts of ethical and religious conflicts.

During sessions devoted partially to combating fears about weight gain, Lonnie is able to construct a family portrait as she experienced it. She speaks about an older brother who frequently turned his athletic prowess into physical aggression against his fearful sister. She experienced an alliance against her on the part of her younger (fourteen-year-old) sister and her brother. And she experienced herself as left out of the family, privy to no important information, confidante to no one, and known by no one.

Two years ago, when Lonnie was fourteen, her mother became severely ill and had to undergo emergency surgery. Lonnie overheard her father talking to his sister on the phone. Her father repeated a statement made by the doctor that it was unlikely his wife would survive the surgery. Lonnie was terrified. Her mother, in fact, made a complete recovery.

During the year of Mrs. G.'s convalescence, Lonnie made herself indispensable to her mother. She organized the household and did most of the housework, while taking care of her mother's personal needs as well. Lonnie increased her prestige in the family, and her difficulties with her brother and sister were eclipsed by her new family role.

Before her mother became ill, Lonnie had been having trouble socially as well. She was a tall girl, nearly five feet seven inches by age twelve, and was nicknamed "Lurch" (referring to a television monster-comedy series) by others in her class. She developed extremely negative feelings about her appearance at this time and became preoccupied with avoiding looking conspicuously unattractive. This sudden criticism of Lonnie's height followed several years of her being referred to as clumsy, because of the visible bruises on her arms and legs. They were from blows inflicted on her by her brother, but she didn't want anyone to know. She sloughed off teachers' and students' questions about the bruises by indicating she had bumped into tables and chairs at home.

Her mother's illness and convalescence provided Lonnie with a legitimate reason to shelter herself at home. She had had fears of abandonment since she was a toddler. On trips, she would never leave her mother's side. Now her mother depended upon her, and it made her feel more loved, less likely to be abandoned. She became obsessive in her desire to offer assistance. She was desperately helpful, thereby, she thought, guaranteeing her place in the family. Lonnie's family noticed none of this drama in their quiet, helpful daughter. While they were aware of her fears about abandonment, they hoped she would outgrow them. None of her feelings of inferiority was ever expressed to anyone. She appeared to need very little from other members of the family.

After her mother's surgery, there was heightened tension

between Lonnie's parents. She believed that her mother blamed her father for her illness, and Lonnie saw herself as "keeping the peace between them." She also believed that she was minimizing friction between her brother and sister by taking blame for grievances they had against each other.

While Lonnie had always stayed as physically close to her mother as possible, she did not feel emotionally close to her. Lonnie felt that neither she nor her mother shared their thoughts or feelings with each other. Nevertheless, Lonnie clung to her mother. Lonnie's relationship with her father was passively critical. She didn't approve of his style of dress or his choice of friends. She complained that he hadn't offered her any verbal or physical affection since she reached puberty. There was a clear demarcation here; when she began to develop breasts, her father promptly ceased being affectionate.

Since her illness, her brother had become increasingly attentive. Though he was away at college, he phoned Lonnie every day at the hospital.

Most of Lonnie's information is given tearfully. She begins each session talking about weight and eating, and requires reassurance before talking about other areas of her life. This reassurance is analogous to a "forbidden meal" that frees Lonnie from obsessing about food and weight. Lonnie, like most anorexics, has had little experience in talking about herself. Talking about her weight becomes a substitute for the kind of introspective talk that most adolescents (though more often girls than boys) engage in.

Lonnie now has to develop a language for herself, where none existed before. She also has to develop a familiarity and comfort with communicating her most personal thoughts about herself. As her therapist, I must take an active role by providing and teaching the necessary vocabulary to Lonnie. Since personal talk didn't occur in Lonnie's household, its very absence suggests that it is forbidden or immoral. (The absence of talk in any area is never regarded as neutral but prohibited or evil.) My task is to counter these negative "taboos of omission" by using specific words and sensitively introducing new areas of discussion. These areas may include verbal coaching in ways of confronting people or expressing anger toward them. In many instances, a positive vocabulary about the emerging, maturing female body must be constructed in order to counter the fears of that body. The responsibility for introducing new vocabulary and the comfortable use of it lies with the therapist. It is only after a trusted person uses previously forbidden words or discusses previously forbidden areas that the patient may follow.

With a patient as childlike as Lonnie, I have the task of developing emotional and reflective concepts so that she can mature mentally to catch up with her body. Though the aim is maturation, it is achieved in a regressive style for a substantial period of time.

In a psychoanalytical therapy, the passive therapist's posture would produce pressure on the patient to reach back and discover important ideas and feelings. In NA therapy, the therapist respects the impoverishment of the patient and provides "emotional teaching" in the way a parent might teach the child basic principles. The therapist's behavior during the course of therapy will change to reflect the growth of the patient. As she acquires and incorporates more mature reflective skills, the therapist gives her more leadership in the process of the therapy.

The evolution of the therapist's behavior during NA therapy is akin to the shifts in parental behavior with a child from age two up to adulthood, now telescoped into the time frame of a three-year course of therapy. The initial goal with an anorexic patient is regression. A major goal is then to move her into adolescence. The threat of adolescence and the implications for separation from parents with whom secure bonds had never been formed terrifies the child, who regards this demand as premature.

The incidences of age-of-onset of anorexia nervosa cluster around two periods in the life cycle of a young person. The first cluster is around menarche and the external physical changes of pubescence. The body seems to be announcing that the dependencies of childhood are officially at an end. Lonnie, like many anorexic girls, was afraid to tell her mother about the onset of her menses for four months. A second cluster forms around the junior and senior years of high school, when going off to college (and the selection of a college) is the task at hand. This time a societally designated separation is impending. The thrust for the early independence of children in our society seems to be producing "masters of isolation" rather than healthy, independent adults. Lonnie is, in her way, trying to master isolation with an obsessive tool—anorexia nervosa.

6

Raphael

Raphael T., a fifteen-year-old boy of extremely high intelligence (IQ 160+), was hospitalized after a ten-month plunge in weight, from 115 to 83 pounds. At five feet six inches, he looked emaciated. He had dark, thick hair, large eyes, and a full mouth, though his emaciated face seemed far too small for his aviator-framed glasses. He stood and walked with a stoop which, paradoxically, gave the impression of an aged person with a youthful skin.

On first encounter, he questions his condition: "I've studied about anorexia nervosa and I know I've got it, but why? This affects mostly girls. I'm not homosexual. Why should I have this illness?" His tone is challenging. It is clear he wants definitive answers. Anyone attempting to assist Raphael will be tested severely as to confidence and knowledge of the subject.

"Who are your role models?" I ask.

He snaps his fingers to indicate that he has discovered the answer to his question. "Of course, I'm a runner. Everything I read tells me to lose weight. All the books on running describe how you're supposed to be thinner than 'other men.' I read one book that said, 'We runners are loners, different and separate from other men even though we are in their midst.'"

Raphael's manner is almost a caricature of authoritativeness. "Okay, so now that I understand how this happened, does that mean I can just make up my mind to get out of this mess?"

"Probably not," I reply in an equally authoritative manner.

"Why not?"

"I think you're overlooking the complexity of the problem. You have invented a way of keeping yourself safe by increasing your running and decreasing your weight. I think you're more committed to it than you've noticed."

He looks pensive. Then he challenges me. "You're saying I can't just give this up?"

"I hope you can, but I don't want you to be disappointed if you can't . . . right away."

"Well, I'm not sure you have the right idea about what I should weigh anyway."

"I think your predieting weight would be fine."

He looks agitated. "I hated who I was then and I'm not going to become *that* again."

"Who were you then?"

"A scared kid whom nobody noticed. I'm very special now because of my running, and I don't want to give that up."

"You'll probably *have* to give that up for a long time."

He looks at me—first with disappointment, then recovering and pointing an index finger. "Why? Why shouldn't I be able to run again? I just won't fall into the same trap."

"Why don't you tell me about this trap? You know, the one you fell into while becoming a runner."

"I kept trying to better my time, increase my distance, decrease my weight. . . ." He grimaces.

I interrupt the silence. "I guess you noticed that at some point your ability to run was diminished by your weakened muscles?"

"Yeah, but most guys are too fat! Do you know what percentage of Americans are overweight? Plenty!"

"Are you mad at me because I criticized you for losing too much weight?"

"I'm just not sure you know what you're talking about."

"You're just not sure that *anyone* knows what he's talking about."

"Yeah, how could you tell? I never think anyone knows much about anything."

He seems relieved. At the end of our meeting, he walks me to the elevator. The elevator doors open. He looks up at me and says quickly in a loud, nervous voice, "What would you do if I went on a one-week hunger strike?"

"Nothing . . . unless your health were jeopardized."

"Then what?"

"A catheter in the chest."

He is familiar with hyperalimentation and points with his index finger toward his own chest.

"Here?"

"Exactly." The elevator doors close.

It was clear from the outset that Raphael was contemptuous of authority. He was disappointed with his parents, whom he was able to manipulate. Each time he succeeded in manipulating them, he felt abandoned. What he brought to his first meeting with me was a set of expectations that I too would fail him—not be his equal, not be competent enough to help him. Raphael, unlike Lonnie, had experienced nurturant behavior, especially on the part of his mother, but he regarded it as impotent nurturance, offering no real protection. It then became the therapist's task to compensate for the impotent nurturance with authoritative nurturance. The former has the quality of being, ironically, dependent nurturance. For very different reasons, Raphael, like Lonnie, never thought it safe to depend on someone else, to trust.

Raphael quickly attempts to take command of the treatment plan by walking out of the hospital two days after my first meeting with him. He telephones me as soon as he arrives home to request and demand simultaneously that I treat him as an outpatient.

"Hi. This is Raphael. I'm home now. I know you don't think that it's smart of me to leave the hospital yet, but I didn't go on any hunger strike, and I want to try it on my own and see you in your office. . . . If it doesn't work and I can't gain weight, or I lose weight, I'll go back to the hospital. Okay?"

Raphael has anticipated any conditions I would want to impose and indicates by that anticipation that he does want to remain in treatment. I accept his well-thought-out plan.

"We'll give it a try. Come in tomorrow at four o'clock."

A male anorexic is atypical. Raphael's acting-out style as well as his outgoing personality is more in keeping with the kind of patient described as the "agitated, manipulative anorexic." Treating the agitated, manipulative patient with NA therapy requires both more authoritative behavior and more structuring than usual. Once a therapeutic alliance has been established, contracts or quasi-contracts with regard to eating, exercising, and weight gain have to be agreed upon.

With the acting-out anorexic, manipulative behavior may take the form of lying, stealing, violence, and wretchedly servile, tearful imploring with respect to weight gain. The last is the most difficult to contend with. A cardinal rule here is that the above behaviors cannot dominate the treatment plan. The patient can be told directly: "While I appreciate your fears, they cannot be in charge. They have controlled you until now and must be resisted so that we can see the strengths that they are obscuring."

All anorexics are dominated by their fears of violating rituals. They rationalize that their strength lies in their ability to follow these rituals. A semantic change, stated by the therapist and repeated often, is necessary. The therapist must help the patient to understand that her or his strength lies in new and independent behavior, and that ritualistic behavior (measuring food, doing a fixed number of exercise motions, counting steps while walking down a hall, and so on) amounts to surrender, signifying weakness and dominance by a destructive set of ideas.

Following are excerpts from the second through the tenth interviews with Raphael.

Raphael enters and glances around the room as if inspecting it, turning his head to focus on each painting and piece of furniture. Then he sits down, arming his face with a self-consciously serious expression. He says nothing.

"So, you like being at home, Raphael?"

He explodes in rapid-fire talk. "It's not that I like being at home. It's just that the hospital wasn't the right place for me. There were lots of doctors there, but they don't *really* understand anorexia nervosa. So what's the point of my staying there? I haven't dropped dead, as you can see. So if I'm not in a medical emergency, there's no reason for me to be in a hospital." He ends on a note of authoritative finality.

"Are you always in charge of yourself?"

"It's not that I *need* to be in charge. I mean, why shouldn't I have something to say about what happens to me? Won't that make me healthier?"

I laugh.

"What's so funny? You think I'm some sort of idiot? I think you should take me seriously!"

"I *do* take you seriously. I also enjoy what a scrapper you are."

Raphael looks confused and voluntarily relinquishes his authoritative posture. "I've calculated that I can eat two thousand calories a day and that will bring my weight up to where I want it. I just don't want to gain too much or too fast. But I want to talk about running. I'd like to go back to it."

"I think you've got running tied in with weight loss,

and that's a strong connection in your head. You don't run reasonably. You run like you diet ... obsessively. Your task is to stop overthinking everything that you do, whether it's running or eating. It's not the act, it's the style, the manner, the overworking of every decision you have to make that's the problem.''

Raphael sinks back in his chair. "You don't think I'll *ever* be able to run again?" His tone is acquiescent, almost pleading.

"I think those strong connections will be with you for a long time, which I will call the foreseeable future. *You* know how strong they are. Running and starving are one idea in your head right now. Why keep yourself in this conflicted area?''

"You don't think that if I set up a *reasonable* goal for a day's running it would be okay?"

"Whether we're talking about running or eating, you rise to the same pitch. Why don't you wait until your weight and eating are under control, and then we'll talk about running?''

"What about bike riding? I've got no intense feelings about that."

"I guess you better buy yourself a bike."

Raphael doesn't compete with me as nurturer but as authority. As his therapist, I have to avoid the threat that Raphael's authoritativeness, and even arrogance, poses. Yet I must also appreciate his need to dominate in order to feel safe. While the compliant patient needs to learn to accept nurturance (which she is offering others continually), the acting-out patient needs to learn acceptance of another's authority. Both patients operate out of distrust of others and a need to control the relationship. One controls by caring for and focusing upon others aggressively, the other with behavior that is more directly authoritative. Many patients use both kinds of behavior to control—behaving aggressively at home, and offering care to others in a passive manner when away from home.

Raphael's acceptance of me as an authority is calming to him in the same way that Lonnie's acceptance of me as a nurturer increases her sense of safety. With each patient, both therapeutic behaviors—nurturant and authoritative—are employed simultaneously, but emphasis is shifted repeatedly to meet the patient's need.

"I keep doing this thing that bothers me. Food is not the only thing I 'overthink,' as you put it. I think about time a lot: how much time I can allocate for studying, for exercising, for guitar playing, for listening to music, for everything. Whenever I'm doing one activity, I'm continually wondering if I should be doing something else instead. I think about how long a time I should spend on it, and I never have any fun because I'm always thinking. I hate thinking!"

"Sounds like you're not able to be spontaneous about much."

"I'm *never* spontaneous. There isn't a shred of spontaneity in my life."

"Are you always checking on yourself?"

"That's what I said before. I have to reexamine everything I do."

"Is that the way you handled your running, and your eating?"

"With running and eating, it felt more like a contest . . . with myself. It even feels like I've lost everything without those contests."

"Have you ever had other contests with yourself?"

"Sort of. When I was in junior high, I used to make up lists. Lists of who I wanted to be my friends, or to like me. I used to keep track of what I said to people, and decided if I said enough 'right' things to get them to like me."

"Did you like them?"

"That was never an issue. I was just trying to figure out where I was . . . socially."

"Not *who* you were?"

"*Who* I was was trying to make it."

"You sound like a production line in a factory. You're always setting goals and quotas in the most personal areas of your life. You talk about how much you do, how much time you spend on it, how well you do it. Do you ever think about fun? Pleasure?"

"I don't even know what that is."

"You're always being too careful to have fun?"

"I have to be careful. If I'm not careful, I could end up like my father. Do you know what kind of business problems he has? He's a disaster! He's a failure! I hate him! He's always telling me or at least trying to tell me what to do, and he's really someone to talk. Do you think he knows how to live? Hah! He's made a mess out of his life. I just get so mad at him. All he does is tell me what's wrong with me. He keeps telling me that *I'm* going to end up in trouble. That's a laugh."

"Has your father always been 'a failure'?"

He is calmer. "No. Just for the last four years. After he left his family's business."

"Have you been careful longer than he's been 'a failure'?"

"Yeah . . . but what he's done just makes it worse."

"So now you have to be doubly careful, obsessive, so you won't make the same mistakes he made?"

"Yeah, I do."

"Sure does sound like a rational strategy."

"You're being sarcastic."

"I think you have to be careful because you can't trust yourself—not your father. I don't think you have ever trusted yourself. I don't think you have any experience with trust or the idea of trust."

"Who should I trust?"

"Me."

"Why?"

"Because you need to learn how to trust."

"How do I know I can trust you? How do I know that you can help me?"

"That's not the issue. The issue in your recovery from anorexia, your lists, your contests, your overthinking— and your loneliness, if you haven't noticed that yet—is your ability to learn to trust."

"Why should I learn to trust you? Why don't I just learn to trust myself? That sounds safer to me."

"Sounds impossible to me."

"Why? Aren't we all supposed to mature into *independent* adults? That means trusting ourselves."

"You can't trust yourself until you have learned to trust someone else."

"How do you know that?"

"Raphael, haven't you been trying to figure out how to trust yourself for most of your life? Isn't that what all your devices, lists, and contests are about? And it hasn't worked. Now you have to use another person to succeed. You've tried it on your own and here you sit. Now try it with someone else."

"You mean I shouldn't trust you on the basis of your trustworthiness but on the basis of my need to learn how to trust?"

"No one could possibly convince you of his trustworthiness, that's the problem. So I invite you to practice on me."

"You *invite* me to trust you?"

"Yes."

"What if it doesn't help?"

"Then you've at least learned how to take a risk."

"You're right! I hate to take risks. I don't like to take chances on anything. I've got to know how something will come out before I start. That reminds me, how long is it going to take before I stop thinking about food and weight so much?"

"That's what I mean. But I'll answer you anyway. I think it will take about a year before it's almost gone, though an echo of it will linger, but without the intensity it has now."

"A year! That's terrible! I can't stand this for another year."

"Your preoccupation with weight will decrease gradually and constantly. Some days you'll have a setback and things will feel worse. You'll have a 'fat attack.' That will happen when something in your life goes badly and your upset becomes channeled into thoughts about eating and weight. The overall pattern will be one of gradually decreasing intensity."

"And all this will happen because I learn to trust you?" Raphael asks sarcastically.

"Yes," I reassure him.

"You're really saying strange things, but maybe you're

right. I just want to ask you one question: How did you know I trusted you?''

After several weeks of outpatient therapy, Raphael begins to act out at home. The faster he gains weight, the more he acts out. His mother phones to tell me that he has become so violent that he is destroying furniture, radios, clocks, everything breakable in the house: "I don't mean to violate the integrity of your relationship, but you must know that we're beginning to fear for our safety and are considering sending Raphael away. Every time he eats and sees that he has gained weight, he throws a temper tantrum—and some furniture."

I explain to Mrs. T. that I will mention her calls when I next meet with her son and that we might consider meeting together with the entire family, including Raphael's older brother, who is no longer living at home.

Raphael's reaction is negative: "I thought that you were *my* therapist—not the whole family's."

I explain that if his family is to become so alarmed at his behavior that they send him to live elsewhere, then he might not be able to meet with me at all. We decide to give it a try.

During the family therapy sessions, Raphael's mother describes herself as worried, even despairing, and frightened over Raphael's behavior. Her husband expresses confusion and anger. Raphael's mother describes concealing her own anger toward Raphael in order to mediate between father and son. Raphael's father describes his efforts to confront Raphael despite the mother's excessive protectiveness. The parents have polarized their own and each other's position when it comes to Raphael.

There is a general consensus that Raphael had emerged early as the dominant member of the family. Raphael denies this, fitfully and tearfully. He becomes agitated and near violent during parts of the first ten meetings with his family. Ironically, he protests violently and aggressively to their exaggerated descriptions of his behavior. His actions during these sessions verify much of their complaints and negate his denials. As therapy progresses, Raphael's behavior is more characterized by sadness and a request that he stop being regarded as the family villain and potential scapegoat for other unhappiness within the family.

The goal of this phase of therapy was to restructure the family members' reactions toward each other as well as their perceptions of Raphael. Raphael's brother, who had played a positive but passive role in the family, began to express his own anger at his father and also at his mother for her role as mediator between son and father. As Raphael's older brother took a more assertive role in the therapy, Raphael became less agitated, and this calmer role in therapy extended to the home. Raphael continued to express anxiety about his increased weight (well within normal limits), but that expression no longer had the violent, aggressive overtones of the recent past.

My role as therapist in the family sessions was typical in that I had to interpret the way each member of the family reacted to the others, the alliances formed and how they functioned, and Raphael's particular place in the family system. Beyond the typical role, I had to maintain my relationship with Raphael. Often, in the midst of a heated discussion, I would act to help Raphael regain control of himself when he was angry and near violence. At other times, I behaved in a coercive way toward Raphael.

"You're so stupid," Raphael says to his father, "how can you expect me to listen to you? I'm leaving! This is a waste of time!" He stands up to leave.

In a firm tone, I tell him, "You can't leave until we have straightened this all out."

Raphael begins to cry. "But we'll never straighten this crazy family out! And I'm *not* such a horrible son! I'm not! I'm not!" He sobs. "I'm not such a bad son."

I then turn to the parents. "Raphael has just listened to twenty minutes of total indictment. It's probably hard for you to hear how thoroughly condemning this sounds to your son."

The therapist is seen not as nonaligned but as someone who shifts alliances continuously during a session in order to protect the overwhelmed members of the family group and to confront the irrational ones. It is an active posture that risks everyone's becoming angry, and is so stated by the therapist in advance: "We will examine what happens between different members of the family, and I will have to referee what goes on here." This offers the family protection from the fears its members may have about their own irrational behavior.

After twenty sessions, Raphael's parents decided that they wanted to enter marital counseling. Raphael was then seen solely in individual therapy. (During the period of family therapy, Raphael was seen twice a week individually as well.) Raphael's comment at the termination of the family therapy sessions was: "When this all started, I always dreaded going home, though I had no other place I wanted to go. Now I even look forward to going home at the end of a day. I'm not sure why it's different, but I'm glad it is."

7

Anorexia Nervosa Combined with Disordered Overeating

Nearly every one of us overeats occasionally, and some make this a regular practice that results in obesity. Recently, a form of overeating sometimes associated with anorexia nervosa and sometimes existing by itself has been noted increasingly by physicians and therapists. Called bulimia, it is characterized by the intake of extremely large quantities of food and liquids, which is then compensated for either by periods of fasting or, more commonly, by self-induced vomiting. While some individuals alternate overeating with extended fasting, most relieve it by vomiting either intermittently, several times during the course of the eating, or at the completion of the eating. The period of time allotted for the eating and vomiting may range from two to five hours or more. The number of calories consumed may exceed ten thousand. The abdominal stretching may result in the participant's resembling a woman in her last months of pregnancy. Data being gathered at present* suggest that between a quarter and a third of all college women interviewed are involved, at various levels, in these disordered overeating practices.

Bulimia (insatiable appetite) frequently accompanies anorexia nervosa. It is distinguishable by the astonishing quantities involved. The bulimic anorexic demonstrates the most bizarre eating behavior in that her swings from overeating and vomiting to stringent dieting or fasting are extreme. If anorexia nervosa represents a desire to achieve safety by overcontrolling eating and weight, then bulimia accompanied by vomiting becomes the safety valve to release the deprivation-spawned rage. The bulimic anorexic began her eating pathology as an emaciated or markedly underweight starver. The starvation produced unbearable stress, which resulted in terrifying overeating episodes.

The act of overeating clashes with the anorexic's need to deny hunger to minimize food intake. When overeating behavior takes hold, resisting eating becomes more difficult. Since eating represents both loss of control and an emotionally intolerable weight gain, and starving becomes harder to sustain, the anorexic is caught in a panic-infused dilemma. Self-induced vomiting seems to resolve the issue. The anorexic surrenders to the urge to eat, even overeat. After she vomits (either at the original suggestion of another anorexic or upon making the discovery herself, out of desperation), she knows she won't gain weight. For many anorexics, only a matter of weeks elapse before they are locked into a cycle of bulimic anorexia. They have alleviated their panic over weight gain but begin to suffer a further loss of self-esteem. They think

*Studies at the University of Chicago and Ohio State have indicated that between 25 and 33 percent of entering freshmen use some degree of self-induced vomiting to control their weight.

self-deprecatory thoughts revolving around their inability to control appetite. The frightening fantasy a young girl may have had about herself as an out-of-control eater has been realized. She carries around a sense of shame that replaces the secret sense of pride she had in her ability to resist food.

The need to keep herself at the lowest possible weight becomes stronger, since it now has to replace the sense of achievement she had about being a highly controlled eater. She sees herself now as chaotic, and becomes almost violent in her eating and vomiting behavior. Both eating and vomiting become clandestine activities. If observed to be eating, yet not gaining weight, she might be suspect. If discovered in the act of vomiting after eating, she would be considered a person who is out of control. She will therefore become secretive and require privacy in increasing degrees. As the overeating escalates and the combined time for eating and vomiting envelops a good part of the day or night, or both, the bulimic anorexic will seek to isolate herself completely. She will disconnect her phone, not make appointments (or chronically break those she makes), and become ever more reclusive insofar as her desires are not socially accepted and she cannot share them with others.

Many anorexics, however, never become bulimic. There is little data at present from which to estimate what proportion of those who began as "starving" anorexics evolved into bulimic anorexics. Yet there are some personality distinctions that can be drawn between bulimic and nonbulimic anorexics. Bulimic anorexics are often more mature socially. They are or have been more outgoing, have had more sexual experience, and tend to run into difficulties with addictive behaviors in the areas of alcohol and drug abuse. Nonbulimic anorexics are wholly invested in "self-overcontrol." They are usually less adventurous sexually and are uncomfortable with the effects of drugs and alcohol. Bulimic anorexics tend more toward addictive behaviors in general. They may smoke cigarettes heavily, whereas the nonbulimic anorexic is more health-food oriented, in many cases, and in a distorted way is seeking a physical purity of body that the bulimic anorexic has forsworn as she gorges herself on sweets.

The bulimic anorexic may run into an even greater number of health risks than the nonbulimic "starver." The frequent vomiting bathes her teeth in hydrochloric acid, which causes gum recession and enamel breakdown. Other side effects and hazards of vomiting are abrasions damaging the esophageal walls, sometimes causing extensive bleeding, and, occasionally, a rupturing of the esophagus, which can be fatal. A condition often found among bulimic anorexics is an abnormally low potassium level in the bloodstream. This potassium deficiency coupled with an insufficient amount of other minerals in the body prevents effective conduction of electrical impulses through the neuromuscular system. An imbalance in these electrolytes can lead to cardiac arhythmias and eventual heart damage. None of these conditions is a function of low weight.

The nonanorexic eating disorder called bulimia/hyperemesis (excessive vomiting) is the newest to be identified and may prove to be the most widespread. Persons within this grouping differ significantly from those with anorexia nervosa or bulimic anorexia. They may have none of the personality disturbances of the former two groups. In fact, they are often individuals who were casually looking for a way to avoid excessive weight gain without giving up excessive eating. Some members of this group were overweight and used vomiting instead of dieting. Some were taught by their friends or athletic coaches or dance teachers this "easy way to keep slim."

Regardless of how one begins this pattern of overeating and self-induced vomiting—whether as a small experiment or out of an intense desire to lower weight—the behavior becomes addictive. Satiety, our ability to appease and satisfy hunger, is altered radically by overeating followed by vomiting. The individual (and in this group men constitute a greater percentage than among anorexics—perhaps 10–15 percent) finds that hunger is abated only after larger and larger meals. Conversely, even if small meals are eaten, a feeling of incompleteness and discomfort intensifies until the individual vomits. Many find that they have become addicted not so much to the large meals but to the vomiting afterwards.

Nearly all those I interviewed stated that they categorized foods in two groups: those foods that did not produce weight gain and could be retained (generally restricted to certain fruits and vegetables) and those foods that had to be thrown up. This latter group included all foods containing sugar, starch, fats, oils—especially cakes, bread, pasta, rice, beef, butter, and cheeses. I have often been told how an individual would eat an "acceptable" meal (retainable category) and then have an "unacceptable" dessert in order to justify vomiting up the entire meal.

It is difficult for most of us who think of vomiting as an uncomfortable and involuntary reaction to severe nausea and abdominal cramps to view it as tolerable and desirable, even pleasurable and addictive. For those who learn to induce vomiting voluntarily, it begins as a necessary unpleasantness and evolves into a sensual, addictive muscular convulsion. No meal feels complete without it. Those who begin vomiting as a diversion come to discover that the behavior they saw as a convenience has wrought emotional and personality changes for them. They begin to suffer the sense of shame and incompetence that the bulimic anorexic experiences. They develop the same physiological syndrome of body disturbances as well. Thoughts of food become as ever present as with the most obsessed anorexic. Other events in the day and evening may begin to take a subordinate place to eating schedules.

The mere fact that an individual is overeating and vomiting is insufficient information for diagnostic purposes. To understand the kind and the extent of difficulty a person is in, it is necessary to examine how this behavior evolved. If the behavior is an attempt to resolve anorexia nervosa, it is a more serious disturbance than if it is the outgrowth of poor dieting habits. The latter does pose serious problems of the type that alcoholism, cigarette smoking, and other addictive behaviors pose. A person's ability to overcome excessive vomiting will depend upon how long she or he has been doing this, how much of the daily routine has been altered to accommodate "the eating," and how much both eating and vomiting have become substitutes for other forms of gratification. (These may include sexual activity, physical activity, socializing, developing and maintaining intimate relationships, and involvement with career and creative pursuits.) Significant additional factors determining the individual's ability to stop the vomiting will depend on general emotional health. Depressed, severely anxious, or otherwise troubled persons will no doubt have a more difficult time extricating themselves from this addictive way of life. Others will have to reorder priorities and return to, or develop, healthier ways to gratify themselves both physically and emotionally. In addition to individual psychotherapy, there are a growing number of group-help programs available to assist those struggling with this type of nonanorexic vomiting behavior.

In the chapters to follow, four women in different stages of life are presented as case studies in their individual efforts to overcome bulimic anorexia nervosa—anorexia that include overeating and vomiting.

8

Amanda

Amanda, a twenty-nine-year-old woman, normally proportioned and rather thin (height five feet four inches, weight 100 pounds), describes herself as a bulimic anorexic. At fifteen, she dieted from a weight of 120 pounds to 92 pounds. She maintained a dieting intake of about five hundred calories per day. While Amanda's weight never plunged to an acute medical risk, most of her recent waking days have been directed by thoughts about food and shopping strategies for obtaining the "right" foods at the lowest prices. For Amanda, the price of food has become almost as important as its caloric value. She has to juggle price, calories, distance from home, and travel time in her scheme of the right way to eat.

Amanda had been diagnosed as "schizophrenic with strong obsessive-compulsive features." She had been hospitalized twice in the past at her own request. She was the younger of two sisters. Her parents, both living, contributed to her expenses (including food). Several years earlier, Amanda had been a highly successful and well-paid writer at an established advertising firm. She was, at the time of our first meeting, working part-time in temporary secretarial positions.

Amanda enters the room, looks around as if assessing impending danger, turns her head in the directions of all four walls and the ceiling, and then takes a seat. She smiles with staring eyes, and in a breathy voice says: "I don't think I like this. This is going to be difficult."

"Do you mean coming here will be difficult?"

Amanda seems lost, disoriented. Her muscles tense, her head is cocked to one side. She is pulling frantically at the skin of her left hand with her right. If allowed to continue, she will become more confused and more frightened.

"Why don't you tell me why you're here?"

She seems too removed to hear the question.

"You were referred by Dr. M. for an eating problem relating to anorexia nervosa, weren't you?"

"Oh yes, although I wouldn't say it was 'relating to' anorexia nervosa. It *is*. I know I don't appear that thin, but I have been thinner and these days I'm eating thousands of calories at a time and spending hours over toilet bowls. I just recently got out of the hospital where I spent three long months so that I could get my bearings. I didn't binge for the entire time but I'm back at it again now." She becomes silent and her face contorts into a smiling mouth and terrified eyes with all the muscular tension visible on the sides of her mouth. Her eyes are unfocused.

"What is happening when your face takes that posture?"

No answer.

"Are you unable to talk? Are you too frightened to talk?"

More silence. Amanda's entire body tenses up. She is holding on to the edge of the chair as one would hold on to a roller-coaster seat, afraid of being thrown off. She stands up, looks right and left for a direction to take, walks around a corner into a hallway, and leans against the wall, out of my sight. I sit there for a minute and then walk to her hiding place. For the next ten minutes, Amanda explains that in addition to having anorexia nervosa, she has been diagnosed as being schizophrenic on two separate occasions spanning a ten-year period. She is concerned that I understand how disturbed she is, and not underrate her state. At the same time, she does not want to be considered less anorexic because of the "second label," as she puts it.

Amanda is unable to initiate talk. My waiting for her to speak disorganizes her, and she spins off into distant and invariably anxious confusion. Here the task is to produce talk continually that is relevant to her and to offer interpretations and explanations for her confused states. It is also necessary to help her understand how therapy might be affecting her on a moment-to-moment basis.

Amanda has two struggles going on simultaneously. She is obsessed with ideas about food and weight, as are all anorexics. At the same time, she is fearful of becoming disorganized, of falling into total mental confusion. Amanda's problems keep the therapist busier than most. Within the nurturant-authoritative perspective, both therapeutic postures may be required in their most extreme form: nurturing behavior to the point of being solicitous, authoritativeness to the point of gentle tyranny.

*   *   *

Amanda returns to the chair and resumes her position on its edge.

"Your facial expression suggests fright and an attempt to conceal it. I don't believe that you know me well enough to be frightened of either therapy or me as a person. Is this a face you use to cope with feelings you have in the presence of your family?"

"They never mentioned my face."

"Are you comfortable with both of your parents?"

"I don't think it's good for me to talk about my parents."

"Why not?"

"They're wonderful people. They're very helpful to me. Talking about them might make this . . . *boring*. I don't want this to become boring."

"Are your parents boring?"

She, becoming tearful, "No. *I* get bored sometimes." She stands up in distress and frustration. "I don't want to feel here the way I do with them. And if we have to talk about them, that's what will happen."

"Please sit down." She returns to her seat. "Does talking about your parents make you feel endangered emotionally?"

"It's something I don't want to do. It's unnecessary."

"Have other therapists asked you to do this? Is your reaction to this topic a result of too many people asking the same questions?"

"No, it has nothing to do with other therapists. It has to do with me. I don't think it serves any purpose except to make me feel like I want to leave."

"I don't want you to leave, and I want us to talk about your parents." At this, she becomes visibly calmer.

* * *

Amanda is able to focus on her mother's strengths as well as implicit demands that she remain not fully competent (or at any rate, remain dependent) in areas of her mother's expertise. She has had to find skills that wouldn't encroach upon or compete with her mother's, whom she has regarded as a "benevolent general." Amanda has always emphasized the benevolent aspect. She found her father to be sympathetic, welcoming her attempts to use him as a role model, which she did. She chose a career nearly identical to his.

Amanda's anorexia nervosa is atypical in that it exists in conjunction with a more severe personality disturbance, schizophrenia. Her thinking is obsessive and always has been. She was an overachiever, like typical anorexics. She attached herself to dieting and being thin with the rigid fanaticism that all anorexics do. Several years of living on five hundred calories a day took their toll on Amanda's stamina and self-discipline. She began to overeat for a period of time, and shifted into a binge-vomiting pattern that lasted ten years. Often, she would break the pattern for several days, and find herself behaving and thinking like a "starving" (nonbulimic) anorexic. She found the feelings of deprivation unbearable, and returned to a pattern of bingeing followed by self-induced vomiting.

In a later session, Amanda refers to an incident where she was responding to a telephone call from her mother— a request that Amanda bring her paprika to complete a recipe. "It was a Sunday morning, and I remember scrambling into my clothes, and rushing out of my apartment. I felt like I was on a critical mission, and was aware of how desperately I wanted to please my mother. I wanted this to be the 'perfect' favor.''

Amanda comes to another session looking brow-beaten. ''My mother made me a sweater. She put a label in it so I could tell the front from the back. She wrote the word 'back' on the label. Wouldn't that insult a five year old? I mean, everyone knows that 'label' means 'back'.''

On another occasion, Amanda walks in looking crest-fallen. ''I called my mother to tell her that I finally found a pair of pants that she wouldn't have to shorten. My mother seemed so disappointed and responded, 'Oh, you know I don't mind doing your tailoring.' ''

Amanda's mother seems to be a fiercely independent woman. On the surface, she appears to be rescuing her daughter at every turn. Amanda has always been offered care by her mother. Praise for Amanda's success in professional achievements is more difficult to come by. When Amanda initiated a research program to study eating disorders, her mother's first comment was, ''Who are you to study eating disorders?'' Amanda's mother is not a villain. She is ashamed to acknowledge the need she has for her daughter. She has made herself indispensable to her daughter instead, and, like an anorexic, desperately takes overly good care of her twenty-nine-year-old daughter so that she won't be abandoned by her. The implicit reversal of dependence between mother and daughter goes undetected as the daughter plays out the externally dependent role. Her mother is sentenced to act out the role of caretaker, for fear her own needs—if directly stated—would not be met.

The following are the foods Amanda eats on a typical binge. The activity of eating, alternating with vomiting (as the abdomen becomes increasingly distended) may go on continually for three to five hours.

Amanda's Typical Binge

2   pounds of vanilla sandwich cookies with vanilla filling
1   pint of vanilla ice milk
1   pint of butter pecan ice cream
2   quarts of skim milk
4   waffles
1   loaf of white bread ⎫
½   pound of butter   ⎬ for French toast
6   eggs   ⎭
1   bottle of maple syrup
1   pound of Ritz crackers
½   pound of potato salad
½   pound of bakery cookies, assorted
a packaged crumb coffee cake (one pound)
2   ice cream sandwiches
2   yogurts
10 cream-filled chocolate cupcakes

This entire binge-vomiting cycle might renew itself after an hour's break. The food would be somewhat different but similar in sugar content. Two such binges in a day were a usual maximum, though occasionally a third followed. After a three-binge day, Amanda would feel completely drained and exhausted for the next two or three days. During a vomiting episode, Amanda would weigh herself until her weight was the same as it had been prior to the start of the overeating. When she returned her weight to that level, she would stop vomiting and go to bed—or begin eating again.

Amanda's obsession had transferred over a period of years from losing weight to maintaining a reasonable, low weight but with as many binges and as much vomiting as possible. Satiety was not determined by how much she ate before stopping. More significantly, it was exhaustion with the whole process of eating and vomiting that dictated the end of a binge. The process at that point was experienced as one behavior. Both eating and vomiting were the two inextricable components comprising "the binge."

"The binge" became an activity that blocked out many other conflicts for Amanda. As a twelve-year-old going through puberty, Amanda was unhappy about the growth of body hair on her arms and legs. She also felt that she was conspicuously chubby. She was hypercritical about her body's proportions. She felt that she was too big "in the middle." One major "unsatisfactory" development she could alter was her weight. She began dieting in the same compulsive fashion she approached other tasks. The dieting enveloped her.

Amanda's bulimic anorexia nervosa had lost much of its compulsivity when I first saw her at the height of her binges—ten years into this behavior. While there were magic rituals that ran through her daily existence, they were not as ever present as in "starving" anorexics. She was seeking a way to stop the binge-vomiting and the financial expense, as well as the shame it engendered. She had emptied her refrigerator and cupboards completely in order to guard against any impulse eating, which might easily escalate to a full-blown binge. She felt it would help to control her eating misbehavior if she telephoned me and reported on it. She brought herself down to two or three binges a week, and then to one. Amanda spent a large part of her sessions discussing the importance of solitude and her great discomfort in the presence of most people. Curiously, Amanda appears to cope extremely well with others. She is exceptionally intelligent and facile conversationally, in a most articulate and often charming manner. Those who deal with her in a work relationship have no indication of her difficulty.

Amanda reached a stage where she wanted very much to scare herself out of going on binges. She sought out a gastroenterologist knowledgeable in the area of bulimic anorexia, and he informed her—with graphic illustrations—of the dangers involved. He described the risk of rupturing the esophagus and the resulting hemorrhaging. She was frightened by this possibility. She used the thought of accidental, self-induced harm to curb the frequency of binges and vomiting and the duration of each episode. In addition, Amanda drew on two of her own experiences as alarming reminders: first, her increasing difficulty in bringing up food; and second, her inability to bring up *any* food on one occasion, which resulted in an emergency-room ordeal that lasted an entire weekend.

For the first year of therapy, Amanda managed to restrict her overeating/vomiting and to cope with the discomfort (as well as the comfort) of intense psychotherapy. She had difficulty with understanding boundaries between therapist and patient and would telephone me several times a week with desperate requests to stop her from eating. Finally, I told her not to call except to change or cancel an appointment, and she was able to handle this limitation.

One day Amanda came in and announced that all binges and especially vomiting were over. "I stood over the toilet and watched a cup of blood run out of my mouth, waiting for it to stop. Or to die. It stopped. I will never do it again."

Amanda remains weight-stable but continues to diet compulsively. When she stopped going on binges, she returned to anorexic obsessing about what to eat or when to eat it. She is still involved in overcontrolling her eating. When dealing with a difficult area in therapy, Amanda may get up and walk over to the mirror to reestablish her appearance in her mind's eye. She then returns to the subject under discussion.

Amanda explains her food-related progress: "I can now coexist with a quart of orange juice and some wheat germ in the apartment. It may not seem like much of a change—and I still pour Ajax on food to stop myself from eating it—but the fact is that I am less terrified of food."

Recovery for Amanda will involve more than giving up compulsive eating patterns. Bulimic anorexia nervosa, with all its dazzling symptoms, is only one in a constellation of disorders that Amanda will have to overcome. If Amanda is seen as a personality in need of construction or consolidation, the therapeutic task becomes helping her to build solidity where there is blank space, chaos, and confusion, all in need of clarification, interpretation, and direction. Nurturing and guiding this growth process becomes very similar to parenting.

9

Adrienne

ACTING-OUT BULIMIC
ANOREXIA NERVOSA

Adrienne walks into the office, sixteen years old, five feet one inch and 62 pounds of uncompromised willfulness. Her entrance has been preceded by a call from a distraught County Director of Social Services, who told me, "If you can't work with her, I'll have to put her in a state hospital. She has already run away from three hospitals—one in the middle of the night in her nightgown. And she never got to the last hospital. While en route, she grabbed the steering wheel of the car as her father was driving, and turned the car onto the highway divider, effectively ending the trip."

Adrienne's appearance is alarming. She is severely emaciated. Her hair is quite thin and her face white. She has an unusual amount of facial and body hair, which she explains she is proud of. Her sleeves are rolled up, and she gestures with her sticklike arms, more to show off their thinness than to augment what she is saying. Her utter defiance of medical reality, the striking clarity with which she reasons, and the energy in both gestures and voice make this marionettelike powerhouse frightening, admirable, humorous, and likable.

She makes it clear from the beginning: "I just want you to know that I like the way I look. I like how thin I am, and I like how much body hair I have."

"And who will make sure that this preferred cosmetic appearance doesn't kill you?"

"The same person who has always made all my decisions for me: Me."

I laugh with friendly amusement. "What do you like best about your appearance, Adrienne?"

"How especially shocking it is to people when they see my arms."

"So, you're a tough guy with skinny arms?"

"Skinny, *hairy* arms."

I laugh again.

"Why are you laughing?"

"There's something humorous about you. Why else would I be laughing?"

She is instantly tearful. "I don't think of myself as funny. Scary, maybe, but not funny."

I grow serious. "Is it important for you to be scary?"

"Well, it's not important for me to *be* scary but to *look* scary."

"How important?"

"More important than anything else. My appearance

is the most important thing in my life . . . except for eating."

"Is eating important?"

"Oh yes. I spend eight to ten hours a day eating. I love how much I can eat and it never affects my appearance." She smiles coyly.

"You spend a lot of time staring at the toilet?"

"Yes, that's easy for me [to regurgitate]. I just drink plenty of liquids."

"Have you always eaten so much?"

"No. I used to eat nearly nothing. For two years I starved. I used to be chubby. I was a chubby eight year old. I always wanted to be thin, and when I was thirteen, I lost the weight."

"Did people around you, your parents, recognize what was happening?"

"Yes. My mother had read about anorexia before I lost any weight, and when I started to lose weight, she took me to the doctor immediately and I was diagnosed. I kept losing weight, and they wanted to put me in the hospital three years ago. My pediatrician panicked. He told me that I would die if I didn't gain weight. According to him, I should have died three years ago. My mother tried to get me to gain weight also, but it was too important to me to give up."

"You make it sound so planned, so deliberate. Did you really have so much choice about this?"

Shyly, she hesitates. "Well . . . I *like* the way I look, but I also feel that I have to look this way. I don't know why, but it's so important to me. I don't know what I'd do if I couldn't look like this." Adrienne quickly becomes tearful.

"How did your father deal with you after you created the auto accident?"

"He yelled at me for a few minutes and then apologized for trying to make me go to a hospital that I hated so much."

"Do you have any experience with compromise?"

"When I want to compromise, I can."

"What about when you don't want to?"

"When I don't want to, I don't."

"Have you ever *had* to compromise?"

"When you say compromise, it makes me upset," she says tearfully. "The only time I ever *had* to do anything was when my parents put me in the first hospital. I stayed there six months and hated every second, until I ran away. It was a waste of time anyway. I can't stand other people telling me what to do. I don't believe anybody really knows what I need better than I do."

"I can see that you have been let down in the past."

"It's not so much that I've been let down. It's just that I don't think anybody knows what I need." She is still weeping.

"Since you're crying so much, I guess you don't have as much confidence as you do authority and control."

"I'm afraid of everybody except my parents. They're afraid of me."

"Are you afraid of me?"

"Well . . . sort of."

"You say you're afraid of me, but it seems to me that you like me."

"Yes, and that scares me."

"Perhaps part of what you like is *not* being in control, being off the case—in here."

"I don't know." She continues to cry.

"Well, I think it would be a good thing if we worked together, but I think it will take quite some time."

"Some time for what?"

"Some time to overcome your problems."

She is crying openly and loudly. "But how do I know we have the same idea about what my problems really are?"

"We don't yet. But we will. I think we will have to knock heads for several years."

She grows calmer. "What if we don't agree?"

"We will have several years to learn how to agree. Unlike the hospitals you have been in, I have one special condition."

"Special condition?"

"Yes. You have to *want* to do this work with me. I only see people who want to work out their problems. No one can be forced to come here. . . . Do you want to do this work?"

"I think so."

"Are you sure?"

"Yes."

"Sometimes we'll disagree, you know."

"That scares me." She begins to cry again. "I don't want to disagree with you."

"Why not?"

"Then you won't like me." She is still crying.

"Disagreeing has nothing to do with liking or disliking."

"It always has for me. I can't stand to disagree with anyone but my parents. I can always disagree with them."

"Is that why you have to be so skinny? Is that why you have to roll up your sleeves and wave your skinny arms at people?"

"I don't know. I just know that I like to shock people."

"I think you like to disagree with people, and that's the only way you know of doing it."

"It doesn't feel like that." She continues to weep.

"We're disagreeing now."

She sobs. "I wish you wouldn't say that."

"We'll have to get better at disagreeing so it doesn't frighten you so much."

"What if I lose more weight?"

"Since no hospital can hold you, I guess it will be up to luck as to whether you survive or not. I would like to weigh you so I have some idea what your chances of survival are."

"You want to weigh me now?"

"Yes."

"What if I don't want to be weighed?"

"You'll have to anyway."

"Why?"

"Because I think it's important. And it's not important for you to battle over that issue."

Docilely, Adrienne stands up and, making a face as if she's been given bad-tasting medicine, walks over and mounts the scale.

"Sixty-two pounds . . . pretty skinny."

Adrienne is smiling proudly. "I bet I'm the skinniest person you work with."

"You just might be. That will add to the accomplishment."

"What do you mean?"

"When you no longer look like this, it will have been a fancier achievement."

"Do we have to talk about that now?"

"No. Now we have to schedule our next appointment."

*   *   *

Adrienne stated her position in her family accurately when she referred to her usually uncompromising posture with regard to her parents. Her parents both experienced themselves as helpless in clashes with their daughter. Adrienne always prevailed. Neither mother nor father could recall an argument in which Adrienne gave in. If she felt she could not control the outcome, violent crying would reduce her parents to compliance. Outside the home, Adrienne behaved in a pleasing, vivacious manner.

Adrienne is the only child of a couple struggling to remain in an upper-middle-class community despite insufficient income. Adrienne's father is an agreeable man who has been depressed since her early childhood and who suffers from visual and tactile hallucinations. Adrienne has learned to accept her father's problems as permanent obstacles to improvement of the family's financial and emotional situation. Adrienne is regarded by both her parents as the happiest part of their otherwise unsatisfying lives. Adrienne experiences no anger with regard to her family's condition. Her only expression of anger is her stated delight in shocking people with her emaciated appearance.

When Adrienne entered therapy, she had been receiving home instruction from her local school district and was spending eight to ten hours a day eating and vomiting. She was spending the rest of her time shopping for food. Much of the family's time and energy were spent in service to the demands of Adrienne's eating schedule. She would harass her father into going back to the grocery store to return "the wrong brand" of a food she had requested. He would comply even if it was late in the evening. A combination of parental fear of her tearful temper and worry that Adrienne might

somehow jeopardize her nutrition further if she didn't get
what she wanted produced total compliance.

Adrienne is used to adults around her reacting to her
fearfully. Her pediatrician "panicked" about her weight, her
parents worry about her constantly. Strangers are shocked by
her emaciated appearance. She has learned to use her illness
to achieve an effect upon people she never anticipated when
first embarking on losing weight three years previously. The
initial consequence of her weight loss was removal from the
ballet classes to which she was so committed. This upset her
and led to a withdrawal from school—and friends. School
officials notified her hapless parents that their daughter should
be in treatment. Adrienne refused.

After reading *The Best Little Girl in the World*, Adrienne
came to therapy with two requirements: that she talk to
someone who would understand her, and that she not be
overpowered or "bossed around." She had spent six months
in a psychiatric hospital before "escaping."

Adrienne's relationship with her family is an example of
one style of nurturing-dependent parenting. Adrienne was
given all that she asked for, and more. Through all the caring
she received, she was aware of a profound neediness and
unhappiness in both her parents. They offered her an intensity
of focus that made her clearly the center of their lives. She
became tyrannical and shared their anxiety if her requests and
needs were not accommodated. She threw temper tantrums
(at home) if things didn't go exactly her way. Her being upset
distressed her parents, so she learned to be afraid of it.

My task with Adrienne is to nurture her and, at the same
time, to teach her to respect her own strengths and to tolerate
compromise and change.

At the time of her fortieth interview, Adrienne has returned to her community high school, and despite her low weight (no gain yet) and drawn appearance, a medical examination shows her to be in satisfactory health. She is doing well in all classes and has been accepted by the other students; several have befriended her.

She enters smiling. "How are you?"

"I'm fine, thanks. What have you been doing and thinking about?"

"I've been thinking that I'd like to study art history when I go to college next year."

"That sounds exciting."

"But I'm worried about something."

"Yes?"

"Well . . . I spend so much time eating that since I've gone back to school, I've had to move it up to late at night. I'm not getting enough sleep, and I don't know how that will work out in college."

"What is your eating schedule?"

"I start at six in the evening, but I don't finish until midnight. I can't begin to do homework until after I finish eating, so I'm starting schoolwork at one in the morning, when I've finished cleaning the kitchen. I have to clean the kitchen myself since I like to know exactly where everything is, and my mother doesn't quite do the job that I do. Actually, *nobody* could do the job I do in the kitchen, and I would have a fit if everything wasn't just right."

"It sounds like it's *your* kitchen."

"Well . . . it is, sort of. You see, I make the family's dinner every night, and that way I can cook extra for myself."

"Does your family mind the way you eat?"

"I don't think they like it, but they're used to it by now. Besides, I'm a good cook, and they're tired after a day's work, so why shouldn't it be *my* kitchen? Anyway," she says more lightly, "my help makes up for the extra expense of the food."

"How much does your eating cost?"

She is embarrassed. "Well, I think it's about a hundred dollars a week—if I'm careful and don't waste much. I mean, I guess it's all wasted, that's what my mother says. But if that's what makes me happy, they'll go along with it."

"So your eating costs *them* money and *you* time?"

She frowns. "You make me sound terrible."

"Is what I said not true?"

"It's true, but the way you say it makes me sound so selfish." She begins to cry.

"You seem so confident and in charge when you're dealing with your parents but so worried about what I say about you."

"Well, I don't want you to think I'm selfish." She is still crying.

"It seems to me that your eating, or this overeating, *is* costly and *does* take up valuable time."

She weeps louder. "Why do you have to keep saying that?"

"Why are you crying so loud?"

"Because what you said makes me feel so bad."

"How do your parents react when you cry this loudly?"

"What do you mean?"

"Do they get angry? Do they get upset?"

"They don't want me to cry." She is still sobbing.

"Then how do they respond to you when you do?"

She sniffles. "My father will generally go along with

anything to stop me from crying. My mother gets upset, but she doesn't give in as fast as my father. She does eventually give in. She's always told me that she loves me and would do anything for me. We have very little money, but I have such good clothes that all my friends think I'm rich. My parents say that's their way of making it up to me for not having enough money so that we could live in a nicer house."

"How do you react to your crying? . . . I'm glad you were able to stop."

"What do you mean?"

"When you start to cry, it's very frantic—the way a baby cries. Then it just keeps getting stronger until you're whining, sobbing, and nearly screaming. Since that's not usual for someone sixteen years old I was wondering if you panic at the idea of becoming upset and then scare yourself when you hear yourself crying."

"Well . . . my parents get so upset when they see me unhappy; I guess it makes my unhappiness seem pretty bad. I don't cry deliberately. But when it happens it gets bad. I don't know why."

"Are you mad at me because I'm not upset by your crying?"

"No, but I get scared when I think you don't understand what something means to me. I think that you won't like me anymore."

"What do you do when someone disagrees with you?"

"I try to avoid it. When my parents disagree, they usually change their minds, but when other people disagree, I get upset. I usually walk away."

"Talking to me must be scary then, since we have an important relationship—sort of like the one you have with your parents, but I don't react the same way they do. I don't want to see you cry, but I'm not upset by your being upset."

"Yes, that does scare me. When I get upset and you don't . . ."

". . . Agree."

"Well . . . yes. Then I get scared of what I told you before, that you won't like me."

"So you have no real experience with argument, especially with people important to you?"

"I guess not." She sounds relieved.

"Then we will be able to practice that here."

"You mean we'll practice arguing?"

"No, we won't make up arguments—we won't 'fake it.' Inevitably, we will disagree on ideas and even decisions concerning your health. When that happens, you will either convince me that you're right, or compromise with me, or settle for a result where we just don't see it the same way."

"But I hate that."

"You hate that because you don't know how to tolerate it yet. I have respect for your ability to learn how to tolerate that even though it will be hard for you."

"But what if I can't do it?"

"You can't do it now, but you'll become able to."

"How do you know that?" She has become tearful again.

"Right now you're doing it—you're crying to change my behavior toward you. I'm not angry with you, but you can't change my opinion about an issue by crying. Anyway, why would you want to win this argument? Winning it would prove you're incapable of change and of growth."

She is crying again. "Well, I don't want to grow up. I really am one of those people who wants to stay a kid. I hate the idea of growing up."

"Why?"

"Growing up is horrible. I'll have to be like the kids who wear all the makeup. I like my body just like it is. I have no shape, no breasts—and I never want them! I don't want any of the things grownups have. Nobody takes care of grownups. You're just on your own. Nobody protects you. I just hate it!"

"I guess you have to argue when you're a grownup. You're not supposed to cry then."

"I don't see why anybody would want to grow up."

"What do you hate most about the idea of growing up?"

"What I just told you."

"Does the possibility of living a life like your parents' scare you?"

"Well, sure. They have less now than they had when I was born. And it looks like it will just get worse, and that's terrible, because when I think that someday they won't be able to take care of me because they'll be too old, I just don't know what I'll do." She is weeping.

"Someday they will be too old to take care of you."

"Don't say that!" She screams.

"I have to say it because it's true."

"But I won't be able to manage."

"Do you think looking young and childlike will prevent your parents from getting older?"

"No, not really. But at least I don't have to act older, and date, and go to parties. Anyway, the thing that's most important aside from school is my eating. So I don't have time to do that other stuff anyway."

"So being younger protects you from adult responsibilities, but it also makes you feel more justified in spending all your time when you're not in school with your parents."

"Well, I like to spend my time at home. I know what's happening at home. I have control over things at home. Everything's organized properly at home. I know what will happen next and how it will happen. I could never eat the way I do anywhere else, and I could never stand to give up the way I eat, so where could I go?"

"You could learn to give up the way you eat, since it's already getting in your way."

"But you don't know how important it is to me! I don't think I could ever give it up."

"I think you could learn to find other ways to make yourself happy. That would make it easier to give it up."

"Why should I have to give it up?"

"For the health reasons we've discussed before, and for financial reasons. There are women who eat the way you do and can't afford it. They spend part of every day stealing from supermarkets. They get stopped, sometimes arrested, but always humiliated."

"I know. That happened to me a few months ago. They caught me with a box of doughnuts and told me never to come into the store again. It's the only supermarket I can walk to, so I have to go there. I try to wait until the manager isn't there before I do my shopping."

"It's already costing you this humiliation then?"

"I still have to do it."

"I want you to scale it down a bit. Cut it to three hours a day from your current six."

"I don't think I can do that." She is crying loudly.

"You don't seem to be refusing me, just crying over the suggestion."

"Well, I'd like to do what you say, but what if I can't?"

"You'll try."

"But what if I can't?"

"We sound like the reverse of *Annie Get Your Gun*."

"How?"

"In *Annie Get Your Gun*, he says, 'No, you can't!' and she says, 'Yes, I can!' Here you say, 'No, I can't!' and I say, 'Yes, you can!' "

Adrienne starts to laugh.

"Then we don't have to be so frightened of your crying or of our disagreeing after all."

"I still don't like it—disagreeing."

"Nobody, or almost nobody, likes disagreeing. We tolerate it and try to resolve our disagreements. Entire relationships don't hinge on every issue discussed between people."

"I guess not."

"You're getting better at it, though."

"Why do I have to learn to disagree?"

"So you can take care of yourself."

Adrienne is in her third month at a college to which she commutes from home at the time of her 130th interview (sixteen months). The daily commute takes nearly two hours each way. She has reduced her eating to three hours a day (3 A.M. to 6 A.M.). She eats nothing during her school day or in the evening. She enters the office looking gaunt and tired.

"You look tired today."

"Yes, I got up late this morning and had to rush

through my eating. I was late for school, but I thought that it was better than not eating at all. I can't believe that I used to do this eating for most of my day. Now I'm attending classes, going to museums, even doing things with other students in the time I used to waste eating."

"That's a wonderful improvement, and one you didn't think you could make."

"It may be an improvement, but I'm falling asleep in class every day and missing important notes. I know that I'm not going to get the grades I've always gotten. I wish I didn't have to do this at all."

"Someday you won't, someday soon."

"I know you think that I can, but don't set any deadlines for me."

"I think it's time you cut this eating out completely, or at least reduced the number of days a week that you do it."

She starts to cry. "I wish you wouldn't say that. I don't know when I'll be able to make further changes in my pattern."

"I think that you'll be able to make them very soon. You should be able to cut down to once a week in the next week or two."

"Don't do that! Don't deadline me!" She is crying louder. "I don't want to disappoint you. I've made a lot of changes already and I can't promise to make more now."

"Just cut down to once a week until you can eliminate it entirely."

Adrienne is crying now and unable to talk. This continues for several minutes while I offer her tissues.

"I know you're having a hard time with this, but what you've already done tells us what you can still do."

"You don't understand. Once I give up the eating then all I've got left is the weight. And next you'll ask me to give that up. I won't! I still like to roll up my sleeves and show people how thin my arms are. I know it's crazy, but I still need to do that, and you *can't* ask me to give that up too."

"I'll ask you to give up everything unhealthy that you're doing to yourself—but not immediately. For now, I think you're ready to give up this eating for at least five of the seven days you're doing it."

"Five of the *six* days I'm doing it. I gave up Sundays two weeks ago."

"You've been getting ready, then?"

"I couldn't have any social life over the weekend, so I don't eat on Sundays."

"That's why you look so gaunt on Mondays?"

"Yes, I don't eat anything on Sundays."

"At last count, you weighed 69½ pounds. Since you're hypometabolic, or 'cheap to feed,' you'll probably maintain your present weight on seven hundred calories a day—or ten calories per pound. Normally, we estimate fifteen calories per pound. I want you to eat seven hundred calories a day, six days a week."

"That means I'll have to go back to measuring calories like I did when I was starving myself."

"That will give us a start. Then we'll bring it up a hundred—"

"No! I'm not ready for that! See, you're rushing the whole thing!"

"I'm not rushing anything. We'll do this gradually until you're ready to give up the skinny arms. You'll need healthier, more direct ways of being assertive than to wave your skinny arms at people to shock them."

"Well, all right. But I'm going to eat on Fridays from now on, and it's going to be a lot to make up for the rest of the week I've given up."

"Fine."

At Adrienne's 140th session (five weeks later), I tell her, "Soon it will be time to give up Fridays."

"I just made such a major change. I don't see how you think I'm ready to give this up entirely."

"I'll be very proud of you when you do."

She begins to cry loudly. "Don't say that. I don't want to think that that's what I'll have to do next. You said that you were proud of me for all the changes I made up to now. This was the worst. Now that I'm only 'eating' once a week and I have to measure the calories on the other six days, I feel like I used to, when I was starving. I spend hours thinking about when I'm going to eat the day's 'rations' and I look in bakery windows the way I did years ago. I feel starved and pathetic."

"When you're able to 'up' your daily intake to about 1,350 a day, that feeling will pass."

"I can't do that! Don't you see? Then I won't look like this anymore. It's very important for me to look like this. It makes people look at me. It makes me special. I don't want to lose that!"

"Look, you've done so many special things already. You go to a top college. You get top grades. You've made friends. You've even been elected to student government. You go to concerts and lectures. You already live a *healthily* special life. Now, you have to give up the only unhealthily 'special' feature of your life."

"I just want to wait a little longer."

* * *

The excerpts from these three interviews were selected to illustrate the confrontations that can occur between therapist and patient. Much has been written about avoiding confrontations with anorexic patients. My experience, however, is that *confrontations within a nurturing relationship* are interactions that affect the core feelings in the anorexic patient. Many anorexics are tyrannical with parents yet throughly intimidated outside of the family. It was important to use Adrienne's trust to help her to take the painful risk of confrontation with the person she had learned to trust. If one facet of the pathology present in anorexia nervosa is passive aggression arising from fear of disapproval of others (excepting parents), then therapy must be the sheltered workshop for the explicit development of the patient's ability to confront another person. The therapist must be supportive of this effort on the part of the patient. What is happening between patient and therapist must be identified continually by the therapist. The very process of therapy must be explained repeatedly to the patient.

Adrienne had learned to see herself as fragile. I had to help her to see herself as able both to change and to tolerate the process of change. The resulting alliance between therapist and patient in this case was strengthened as each confrontation and its accompanying change was negotiated. Adrienne learned from therapy that she was more powerful, and more flexible, than she had believed. She learned to trust and depend on another person—and herself—in the process.

10

Jeremie

LATE-ONSET ANOREXIA NERVOSA

Jeremie, a woman of forty-six, is thin, verging on emaciated. She has three daughters—thirteen, eighteen, and twenty-five. She has been married for twenty-seven years to a successful oral surgeon. Jeremie developed anorexia nervosa in her early forties and has been struggling with it for four years. In the initial meeting, anorexia was referred to only peripherally. Jeremie's main concern was abdominal pain, which she claimed was relieved only by vomiting. Extensive examination by several gastroenterologists produced no positive findings.

A smartly dressed woman, Jeremie enters the room and asks, "Who sits in which chair?" Her manner is friendly and nearly humorous.

"I sit in the one that swivels and rolls. You can have any other."

Her next remark comes quickly: "This is probably not as skinny as some, but it's my worst. What do you do when every time you eat, you get terrible pains in your stomach and nothing can make them go away until you throw up?"

"Have you seen physicians about this?"

"Yes. They all called it 'head pain.' So here I am."

"You sound reluctant about being here."

"I don't think this can hurt me, in any case. I'm just not sure that something couldn't be done medically for it, but I'm getting tired of all the tests and eventually could be damaged by some of the more invasive ones."

"Does that mean you're here because you think the pain *is* caused by emotional distress—or because the physicians have given up on you?"

She laughs. "I guess I should have decided why I'm here. I've got plenty of head pain that I *know* is head pain and this," she points to her abdomen, "will have to wait."

"Your style is to stay in charge of your own case, whether medically or psychiatrically?"

"When you're married to an oral surgeon, you get to know too much to be passive about your own medical care."

"Do you know too much about psychology and psychiatry to let someone else be in charge of your psychotherapy?"

"Do I sound like I'm trying to be in charge here?"

"You sound like it's scary *not* to be in charge anywhere."

"When you bring up three children, you learn how to be in charge, or they're in trouble."

"Are there other people that you're in charge of, in addition to your children?"

She laughs and rolls her eyes. "Is there anyone that I'm *not* in charge of?"

"Could you tell me who else that includes? Your parents? Your in-laws?"

"My parents means my mother, and nobody could be in charge of her. My mother-in-law is self-sufficient."

"Do you feel like you're in charge of your husband?"

"Responsible for . . . but not in charge of."

"Is that good?"

"*He's* good, but he also is well taken care of."

"So far you've told me about being a surgeon's wife, being in charge of your family. But how does this affect you?"

She laughs. "Don't ask."

"But I *am* asking. And it's apparent that it's difficult for you to tell me. Do you tell anyone?"

"What's the question?"

"Do you tell anyone how your life affects you?"

"I tell my friends about my kids. They tell me about theirs." There are a few moments of silence. "Is that what you mean?"

"Telling your friends about your kids isn't telling them about *you*."

"Sure it is. That's the most important part of me."

"Jeremie's an unusual name for a woman."

"Spelled 'i, e,' but I think you're right. There's no such name for a woman, that I know of anyway. My mother just wasn't accepting anything less than a boy."

"*Less* than a boy?"

"She didn't touch me until she had to leave the hospital. She had a boy's name picked out and anyone who came along got it."

"You're smiling. Does that mean you're angry?"

"It's too late to be angry about that. It *is* a pain in the neck, though, when I order something on the phone and I tell them my name and they assume it's my husband's. The poor guy gets mail addressed to Dr. Jeremie—all the time.''

"It seems to me it's the 'poor woman' who gets no mail. You never got to tell me whether that annoys you."

"You get used to it."

"Did it *ever* annoy you?"

"It's funny, when you think about it."

"Is it always funny?"

"I don't always think about it."

"What would you like to happen here?"

"Whatever is supposed to happen here."

"I mean, what are your goals for therapy?"

"To get rid of this 'head pain.' "

"Aside from the physical relief from your stomachache, do you have other goals, feelings you'd like to resolve?"

"If they'll help get rid of this pain."

"It's going to be difficult to get rid of that 'head pain,' as you call it. The first idea that you'll need to get used to is that you're in treatment for an emotional disorder that has resulted in your needing to be unhealthily thin. This is part of a group of irrational ideas resulting in near emaciation, abdominal pain, and an inability to respond to any questions about your feelings. It's apparent that you're a 'good trouper' and that you can take a lot of punishment without complaining or even admitting that you're hurting. To some degree that's admirable; beyond a certain point, it becomes what we call 'denial.'

" 'Denial' plays a lot of tricks on your mind and your body as well," I continue. "Not knowing what you're feeling about yourself and your life is like not being able to sense physical pain. You can't tell if you're injured, cut, scraped, burned, broken, or bleeding. Psychologically, you may be all of these things. You and I need to survey the damage. I will be asking you all sorts of direct questions about feelings. If you don't answer, then I'll ask them again—not because I'm annoyed, but because you seem to have no experience in talking about yourself. We will have to develop a language for you so that you won't need to deflect all personal questions and continue to use this 'denial' thing I've been talking about.''

"You certainly don't beat around the bush, do you?"

"If I'm not direct, we will have many pleasant, cheery chats here, and you'll be thoroughly neglected in the process. Are you good at getting yourself neglected?"

"The best. . . . Was that a good answer?"

"That was a good answer."

Adolescents suffering from anorexia nervosa often indicate a need to be in charge of themselves to an inappropriate degree. They also feel safer, though contemptuous, when in charge of authority figures around them. Jeremie is at a point in her life when her inappropriate needs look appropriate. She is a mother in charge of her children, and a wife in charge of her household. Whereas adolescent anorexics don't have the outright credentials to mother or nurture those around them, a mature mother of three may act in an overly nurturing manner solely to receive more praise for it. She may be doing this out of the same fearful mistrust as the teenage anorexic—specifically, that if she doesn't provide an abundance of care for those around her, they will not value her.

The NA therapist's task in doing regressive therapy with a mature, sophisticated patient is more complex and is best achieved by enlisting the patient's collaboration. This is done by making the process of psychotherapy explicit on a session-by-session basis. By analyzing *what* is happening between the two persons involved in the therapy, the patient gradually relinquishes her defensive posture. The therapist states goals repeatedly and the patient participates in the process. The goal of the regression is the same as for the adolescent: the development of extraordinary trust. The ways of attaining it are more fully spelled out and in that way ensure the self-esteem of the patient, who self-consciously permits this regressing relationship to develop.

"Are we going to find out why I have this head pain?"

"We already know why you have the head pain. We want to help you find new ways of dealing with yourself that will help you eliminate the side effect of head pain."

"Are you going to ask me about my childhood?"

"We will need to collect historical information about you so that who you have become will make more sense to you. Most people think that the information, or finding the right information, is the cure. Actually, it's the *process* that's therapeutic. The information found and the questions designed to find it are merely vehicles that allow us to relate in a way that will be helpful to you."

She says nervously, "What way of relating here will be helpful to me?"

"You, using me as a helping person."

"Sounds like you want to be my mother."

"Was your mother a helping person?"

She pauses. "*I'm* a helping person."

"Then *I* want to be *you*."

"Then you want to be the mother I wish I had."

"Are *you* the mother you wish you had?"

"To everyone but myself."

"Do you allow anyone to take that role with you?"

"Nobody has ever tried . . . and probably no one could handle it."

"Why not?"

"They'd fall apart from the effort."

"Who'd fall apart from the effort?"

"All of them."

"Who are we talking about?"

"My mother, my husband . . . and I wouldn't ask that of my kids."

"Have you ever played the *supported* role in a relationship?"

"People aren't comfortable being supportive."

"Is it possible that you're frightened of receiving support in a relationship?"

She responds in a subdued tone. "Are you saying it's my fault?"

"I'm suggesting that you're frightened. It's not your *fault* if you're frightened."

"If I'm frightened, then there's something wrong with me."

"You seem to take responsibility for yourself and everyone around you."

"Isn't that what a 'mommy' is supposed to do?"

"Is that what your 'mommy' did?"

"She would have, probably, if I'd let her."

"So you also take responsibility for your mother as well as for your husband and your children?"

"If I'd been a different kid, I probably would have gotten what I wanted."

"Which one of your children has had responsibility for your treatment of her?"

"None of them." She shakes her head.

"Do you feel guilty toward your mother?"

"If I knew how to deal with her, she would have said kinder things to me."

"So, you use responsibility to avoid feeling helpless."

"What do you mean?"

"As long as you can feel responsible toward everyone, you can always blame yourself for what goes wrong. And you never have to feel at the mercy of anyone else's feelings or behavior. It's easier to say 'I was in charge and I blew it' rather than 'I was the victim of someone else.' It's the possibility of being the victim that scares you, so if you always blame yourself you can't ever see yourself as someone else's victim."

"Why would I be so worried about being someone's victim? . . . Is that why I don't know when someone insults me until several days later?"

"That's part of it."

"What's the other part?"

"If you don't notice when someone hurts you until a day later, you don't have to confront him or her. The next day you can believe that it's too late anyway, so why bother."

"That's true. I can't confront anyone about anything personal."

"You're afraid they won't like you anymore?"

"Probably."

"And it will be your fault if they stop liking you?"

She smiles. "I'm in great shape. I'm scared of feeling helpless or disliked, and I can't accept anyone's care."

"Should I throw you in the garbage now?"

"Am I going to find out worse things about myself?"

"What do you expect to find out?"

She is concealing tearfulness. "I've always been afraid . . ." She looks at the floor and slows to a halting whisper. ". . . That I'm going to find out there's something terribly wrong with my character, something bad enough to drive everyone away."

"I think that you'll find out what you already know."

"What do you mean?"

"That you've always been afraid."

"Of what?"

"We could call it fear of abandonment—by everyone— or call it a nameless terror."

"It hasn't always been so nameless."

"What forms has it taken?"

"When I was a child, I was afraid to drive across bridges in cars unless a man was at the wheel."

"Did your father drive?"

"My father died when I was two."

"Did you feel bad about not having a father?"

"I'm not even sure. It's just the way it was."

"Were there other fears?"

"Fears of heights, even fears about going out of the house at one point. I used to be terrified of flying, but I've got that down to a fear manageable with two tranquilizers." She laughs.

"When you talk about all these fears, you don't allow yourself much expressiveness. It sounds like you're describing someone else."

"I don't like to relinquish control."

"We'll have to make that a major goal here."

"Good luck." She laughs again.

At the time of her eightieth session (fortieth week), Jeremie has made a strenuous effort to reduce vomiting to twice a week, depending upon stress. She is viewing it as a stress reaction and has experimented with new behavior toward her family that helps reduce "nameless terror." Anticipating the changes in behavior has increased her fears, but implementing them has calmed her. The nature of the changes follows the theme of encouraging each member of the family to assume a greater responsibility in the house. Everyone has to hang up his and her own clothing. Jeremie has let go of the job of picking up after four members of the household.

Jeremie had structured the family in a manner that made her indispensable. She did everything for everyone. Jeremie trained them to expect service that she resented giving. She has come to realize that she feels safest when she is the most needed, but she is fearful of not being needed enough. While there was some initial resentment on the part of those who experienced reduced service, the reduction was not severe and everybody in the family has proved able to adjust.

"I'm getting better at asking for what I want and refusing what I don't want. Do you think it would be worthwhile, or more worthwhile, if I came three times a week instead of two?"

"Do you want to come three times a week?"

"If it would make a difference."

"Your asking for that *is* a difference. Yes, I think you should get what you want."

"Why do you answer that way?"

"I'm emphasizing what is happening here. I'm deliberately keeping my response in the form of acceding to your request rather than making a mechanical decision to do 'the right thing.'"

"But would it be better?"

"Is this something you want to do?"

"All right." She smiles. "I get the point. Yes, 'mommy,' I would like to meet three times a week."

"You're joking to avoid expressing sincerity."

"Oh, you're getting 'direct' again."

"And you're *not*. Why?"

"You know this is very difficult for me. I have enough trouble with the guilt I feel about spending time in something as selfish as this."

"Then why *are* you coming here?"

"I can see that it's helping my family."

"We could probably help your family more by having them come here and you stay home."

"Okay! It's helping *me*!"

"Do you understand why that's so hard to say?"

"I feel I shouldn't need help. I have a good life. I have no reason to have problems. I know that's not true, but part of me still believes it, and that's the part of me that makes me feel guilty and selfish. It's also the part of me that feels there is still a terrible part of me we haven't discovered, but will."

"How do you protect yourself from people discovering that part of you?"

"I never sit still. I work as hard as I can, as long as I

can. Sitting still is a terror. If I'm working, no one can accuse me.''

"Who actually does accuse you?"

"Me."

"Where did you learn to accuse yourself?"

"I accused myself long before anyone else could."

"Who could?"

"My mother often did, but I always thought and often still think it was my fault. If I knew how to handle her, she could say those things to me."

"Who is responsible for how you're treated here, whether you get better or not?"

"I am, I guess."

"Who would be responsible if someone came to your husband for oral surgery and that patient lost the tooth?"

"If it could be saved, my husband would save it." She laughs.

"Who would your husband consider responsible?"

"Himself."

"Who do you consider responsible if your children have problems?"

"Me."

"Who do I consider responsible if my patient shows no improvement?"

"Oh, that's different."

"Why?"

"Because I—"

"Because *you* are the patient?"

"I guess so."

"So *you* are responsible for the whole world, but no one is responsible for you? It's a good deal for the rest

of us but not for you. Are you still afraid to see yourself
as dependent, trusting? Does it still mean helplessness?''

"I think you're tougher than my mother."

"Do I have more responsibility for you than she
had?"

"Wow! All right. . . . That hit home."

"The issue is no longer your mother. The issue is the
rest of us in your adult life."

She says, softly and slowly, "Do you think I'll ever
get over this? Don't you think I'm too old for this? This
is a kid's disease, and it's hard enough for them to
overcome it. I'm in my forties."

"If I live up to my professional responsibility to you,
you should overcome this."

"Aren't you setting a tall order for yourself?"

"You came in here with the fear of gaining weight and
the stomach pains. Reliable physicians have stated that
you suffer from 'head pain,' so it's my responsibility to
work with you to get rid of this pain. I think you're a
resourceful person, and I have to take responsibility for
that estimation too."

"Can you get everyone over this?"

"No."

"Why me?"

"That's the way I see it."

"I hope you're right."

"I think you believe I am, Jeremie."

"So, I guess you're going to be my mother—and
father—for the next few years."

Jeremie's last remark, which shows her acceptance of the
therapist as a parent figure, is said with surprising frankness.
Her resistance to indicating or declaring directly that a trust-

ing relationship exists suggests how uncomfortable it is for Jeremie to see herself as a person being helped. It is as if it is an immoral position. It is also a frightening situation to be in.

Jeremie associates being a helper with safety and power. Depending upon others for help is experienced as being vulnerable, endangered, and powerless. To depend upon another is to trust where there is no expectation of reliability. She is safe in the role of mother and does not find a mothering role with her husband uncomfortable. She happily comments that her husband couldn't handle a relationship that would call upon him to be more supportive. They have both nurtured this idea about him throughout their marriage. This has resulted in a situation in which Jeremie has "structured out" anyone's ability to act supportively toward her. In fact, no one in her family could have conceived of Jeremie as a person needing emotional support at any time.

Jeremie experienced her relationship with her mother as ne in which she fearfully pleased her. She saw her mother as eeding a great deal, being able to offer very little, and being urious when disappointed. Jeremie quickly and almost instinctively learned to please everyone around her. When they were pleased, they would not criticize or abandon her. Pleasing others became her way of "controlling" them, of protecting herself from fears of potential aggression against her. What appeared to others as a delightful trait borne of security, this "people pleasing" was seen by Jeremie as her only protection and even her weapon against mistreatment and neglect. In therapy, this was explained to Jeremie explicitly so that her behavior in the therapeutic sessions could be understood as resistance to receiving help and fearfulness over giving up the safety of the helper role.

One of Jeremie's defenses against revising her relationship with her family in the direction of a more assertive, less pleasing posture was her fear that others in the family would be damaged by such a change. During the previous year, several members of her family had been briefly, though seriously, ill, and required short-term hospitalizations. She saw her family as a permanently vulnerable group who would always need excessive care. Once this was identified as an invention to forestall change on her part, she was able to relinquish it by degrees. While many anorexics develop anorexia nervosa at the time they first face separation from their parents, Jeremie developed anorexia when she saw her family begin to leave home for college and adult life.

11

Sarah

Sarah is twenty-six, married five years to a physician. They have two children, a girl aged two and a boy three. Sarah developed anorexia nervosa at the age of twenty-one. A year later, she was hospitalized and "learned to vomit" from another anorexic patient. For the past four years, Sarah has been a severely bulimic anorexic, given to spending much time eating and vomiting. Initially, Sarah described herself as withdrawn, angry, and out of control. Her appearance is emaciated; she is five feet five inches and weighs eighty-four pounds. She has a large frame, which makes her look thinner. She feels that her appearance is reasonable, though she understands that family and friends think her too thin. She sympathizes with their point of view and wants to see herself as too thin but is unable to. Her limbs are bluish due to the appearance of veins under the skin surface. She has excessive

117

body hair since losing weight, and her parotids (the glands at the base of the jawbone) are severely swollen.

"I hate the way I look, but it's not my weight. It's my swollen, chipmunk face. When I got married, I was pretty. I didn't always look like this."

"Did you like looking pretty?"

There is a silence. "No. It's just trouble. I was always told that if I looked too pretty, I would be asking for it."

"Asking for what?"

"Asking for trouble from men. . . . You know . . . assaulted, hassled."

"Do you want your husband to find you attractive?"

"My husband hasn't found me attractive since the day that we were married."

"Did he tell you that?"

"He told me that he didn't like the way I looked, and I was a normal weight then. He was critical about the physical aspect of my femininity. I didn't know whether I was physically inferior to other women or whether we were all really disgusting to men. He made me feel like I was repulsive. I tried to be more acceptable but finally gave up after the first year of our marriage. I thought that if I lost weight, maybe that would help. That message was in all the magazines, all the newspaper ads. I just thought it might help. I began to lose weight and, like everybody else I've read about, I got trapped in it. I hated the starving, but it was the only way to keep the weight down. Then I found out about vomiting. After that, eating, instead of starving, became most of my life. If it weren't for my children, I wouldn't even want to give it up. I love them and they need more mothering time. I postpone this till after they fall asleep, but I'm so weak I have trouble carrying them around. They're both in diapers, so weak is the last thing I can afford to be."

"How could you conceive the children at this low weight?"

"My weight varied. When it went up I got pregnant . . . during the few times I could drag my husband into bed." Her tone is sarcastic. Suddenly she bursts into tears. "Can I get over this? I don't want to be like this the rest of my life. I'd rather die than go on like this. If I didn't love my children so much, I'd give up on everything."

"If you want to overcome this, you will."

"Do I have a chance?"

"Yes, more than a chance."

Patient morale is important in overcoming anorexia nervosa. A level of confidence in the therapist that would be considered unhealthy and undesirable in a more analytically oriented approach is necessary in NA therapy. The development of extraordinary trust in the therapist as an active agent in problem solving must occur if the patient is to exchange rigid, obsessive behavior and thinking for flexible, healthy behavior. It is this trust for the therapist (eventually transferred back to the patient) that tempers and eliminates obsessive patterns.

After Sarah has had three weeks in treatment (twice a week), her husband telephones. He says that his wife is in a clinically catatonic state, and that she has not been able or willing to talk or move for two hours. I ask him to bring her to the phone. He attempts to talk her into coming to the phone. She doesn't respond. I ask him to carry her to the phone and hold the phone to her ear. He does so.

"Sarah, can you hear me?"

There is no response.

"If you can hear me, say yes."

"Yes." This is said stiffly, with an obviously clenched jaw.

"Can you tell me what you're upset about?"

"No. Can't talk."

"Can you move your arms?"

"No."

"Now try to move your fingers on your right hand. . . . Can you?"

"Yes. Little."

"Now move the fingers of your left hand."

"Yes."

"Now, I want you to move your entire right hand so that it's raised."

"Hard."

"Try again."

"Can do but hard."

Her speech remains primitive but begins to loosen up as she becomes able to move more freely physically. The process takes a half hour. She later reports that it actually required several hours for her to move and speak normally again. The incident followed an argument with her husband concerning the amount of money he would give her to manage the household.

Sarah was the youngest of three daughters. She experienced her role in the family as the least powerful. She lost all arguments to her mother and sisters. She was considered attractive but was admonished for it, lest she get into trouble.

She did well in school and thought about becoming a dentist like her father but was told by him to become a dental hygienist. She did so, and used her talents to support herself and her husband while he was attending medical school. She was attracted to her husband because of his mild manner and his "lack of sexual pushiness." She met him several months after being raped by a member of the college faculty—an incident that verified her mother's warning about displaying attractiveness. She felt ashamed, blamed herself, and never reported the crime. Sarah blamed herself for whatever befell her, especially for the behavior of others directed against her. She found it difficult to get angry over personal encounters. Sarah accepted blame for the rape episode until she began to talk about it for the first time.

After two months in outpatient treatment, Sarah asks to be hospitalized. She feels that she will need a more supportive environment in order to give up the overeating, vomiting, and low weight. She is admitted to a hospital, on a medical floor, and is counseled daily by a sensitive internist as well as the hospital dietitian. Sarah stops vomiting as soon as she enters the hospital. She picks at her food as she had done as a "starver."

"I can't throw up here. It's not private enough. I'm happy about that, but now I'm scared that I'll eat the way I did three years ago."

"Why don't you start with a daily intake that will maintain this weight?"

"I've lost touch with caloric reality. I don't feel I can determine what will maintain my weight."

"Can you trust people in the hospital like Dr. Blank and the dietitian to give you the right amount?"

"I think I can trust them. What do you think?"

"I trust them. That's why I work with them."

"I guess if you can trust them, so can I."

"Aside from my trusting them, what are your own impressions?"

"They're interested, and they seem like they care. All right, tomorrow I'll start eating. This whole thing is so crazy. I can't believe that after eating ten thousand calories a day, I'm afraid to eat eight hundred. It does feel good not to vomit, though. Will I ever find some sane middle ground? I mean, do I have to eat either thousands of calories a day or starve myself?" She is tearfully annoyed with herself.

"You always seem so annoyed with yourself."

"What else could I be? I'm a grown woman with children and responsibilities, sitting here in the hospital while my mother takes care of my children because I'm too crazy to know how to eat normally. I'm still afraid to be an average weight since that looks too fat to me." She points to her thighs. "Of course I'm annoyed with myself. I'm a disgrace." She starts to cry.

Over the next three weeks, Sarah gains four pounds. She continues to eat without vomiting. Most of the talk is addressed to the issue of self-blame. She has blamed herself for not being as good or as smart as her sisters. She blames herself for not having been attractive enough to her husband, and she blames herself for not achieving a higher career level. She makes a connection between not wanting to gain weight and not wanting to be a "temptation" to men. She discusses the rape incident but apologizes for it throughout her narrative.

"When it was all over and I was crying, he looked at

me as he was walking away and said, 'What's the big deal anyway?' "

"Did you think it was a 'big deal'?"

"I thought it was a big, stupid mistake."

"Mistake?"

"Yes. If I hadn't agreed to talk with him at his home instead of at his campus office, I wouldn't have set this up."

"Was it your idea to meet him at his home?"

"No. I gave him my schedule, and he said that he didn't have any conference time available during my free time, but that he could meet with me at his home. He sounded so professional, but I should have been smart enough to figure that out."

"Do you believe that you provoked a sexual assault?"

"By going to his house, I provoked anything that happened."

"What did happen?"

"I was sitting in his living room. I had brought a first draft of my paper, and put it on the coffee table. He said he had to wash up or something, and left the room. He returned several minutes later, and told me to get undressed. I thought he was kidding. I laughed and nervously said that I thought we would talk about my paper. He said 'After.' I didn't really believe it, but he seemed to rip off my clothing while I sat still." She becomes severely agitated, and begins to cry intensely. "I never told anyone before. I sound too stupid. I must have worn the wrong clothing! I must have said something wrong! He was a member of the faculty. If he were a rapist, someone would have had him arrested. Do you think that I'm awful? That I'm a . . ."

"A whore?"

"Yes, dammit—a whore! A whore!" She is crying intensely.

"Of course you're not a whore. You never were. What you were was a naive college freshman who was victimized by a faculty member. You're also suffering from a case of what I call 'impotent overresponsibility.' "

"What do you mean?"

"You felt powerless at home but responsible for everyone's behavior and judgments relating to you. Then you went away to college and felt powerless yet responsible for being raped. You keep accusing yourself of doing the wrong thing. Whatever happens, you blame yourself. It seems you so distrust yourself that you can't even distinguish those times when you're really helpless from times when you can influence events affecting your life. At any given moment, you feel simultaneously powerless and all-powerful. The only area where you can comfortably, if not desperately, act exclusively all-powerful is in keeping yourself emaciated. And emaciation is the safest state, since you always feel the impending danger of becoming powerless to control your appetite, and ultimately obese. It's much too frightening for you to feel helpless, so you blame yourself for being raped. Then you can feel guilty about it. But that's better than feeling helpless about it—that's the worst choice of all."

"You mean that it wasn't my fault?"

"Here we would have to say that 'fault' in the way you're using it implies conscious choice. Did you have an awareness at the time that by going to your professor's home you were taking a fair risk of being raped?"

"No. I never thought about the possibility."

"Then you never *decided* to risk being raped. You had not chosen. There was no choice, therefore no fault."

Sarah looks confused, then relieved. "How do I know when I have a choice or not?"

"When you *feel* like you have a choice. Right now, you don't feel like you have much choice about anything. Our task is to build areas where you have choice, and expand them. The two areas we will start with are self-assertiveness and eating. The first has to do with choice with regard to others; the second, flexibility in behavior—especially eating and weight, which only affects you. Unlike angry adolescents with anorexia nervosa, you aren't holding your body hostage against your parents. Your weight control is more self-directed. You are afraid of what men may do to you if you present an attractive appearance—but that's probably secondary to the issue of self-control."

"How do I work on these areas?"

"I want to give you assignments in both areas. During the week, at different times people here in the hospital will inadvertently not do for you what they were supposed to. Others will get on your nerves. Your homework is to find a way to express your displeasure."

"But I don't want to get into fights with people."

"I'm not talking about getting into fights, or even strong arguments. We have a language filled with terms of moderate discontent. For example, you can use phrases like 'I am disappointed with . . . ,' 'I am uncomfortable about . . . ,' 'I am annoyed with . . . ,' 'I would rather you didn't. . . .' None of these is murderous in nature. None of these threatens lifetime friendships. They are just mild indicators of our displeasure. If we didn't have them in our language, we would all have to be mind readers or live in constant fear of the unexpressed pain we might cause others.''

''What's the second homework assignment?''

''That's just as difficult. I want you to deal with your eating and weight in a self-conscious, reflective way at each meal. Ask yourself why you have to overcontrol your weight. Try to separate attractiveness from provocation of being raped. Since you see yourself as unattractive at this weight, examine the choice of becoming more attractive. Do this while sitting with your meal in front of you. I'm not asking you to gain weight at this point, just to understand the constriction you experience over eating.''

''That one sounds harder.''

''Do you still feel responsible for being raped?''

''No. For the first time in eight years, I don't.''

''Would you like to feel that sort of 'pardon' about starving and being emaciated as well?''

''Is that possible?''

''Do you want that?''

''Yes, of course.''

''Then that's the goal.''

Sarah, as a more mature and healthier anorexic, can be dealt with on a more rational level than a frantic adolescent. Sarah has more circumspection, and that can be put to use to expedite recovery. The structure of a nurturant-authoritative approach is still there, but Sarah can handle more insight work.

Sarah returned to her home after six weeks of hospitalization. She gained eight pounds and gave up vomiting as well as overeating. After two months, she began to overeat and vomit two to three times a week. Much of this was due to stress related to mothering two children still in diapers and to difficulties with her husband. Within a month of resuming this bulimic anorexic pattern, Sarah relinquished it entirely. She made a commitment to herself to deal with stress in healthier ways. She became more assertive and reorganized her daily life to have more time to spend with other adults. Her swollen glands went down and she began to enjoy her increased attractiveness. In the sessions following the initial mention of the rape, Sarah expressed a need for permission to become angry at the perpetrator. She used this permission to free herself from feelings of guilt, and fear of becoming attractive. Today, she still does some minimal controlling of her eating and weight, but it is well within what is considered normal. As Sarah puts it, "I won't say I don't care at all about my weight and eating, but not much, and not obsessively."

Sarah, appropriately, seeks as her main objectives to develop relationships with friends, to build her self-confidence, and to increase her flexibility as well as to resolve problems in her marriage.

12

A Summary of
Treatment Strategies

A therapeutic approach that is both nurturing and authoritative allows for variation in order to accommodate the needs of patients seemingly homogeneous, but within the sameness differing in degree of pathology, maturity, age, sex, availability of supportive people, and stability of environment.

The six individuals discussed in the preceding chapters illustrate some of these differences. Their symptoms vary within a pattern. Externally, each person began dieting and became enveloped by the syndrome of anorexia nervosa. They all discovered ways to utilize the trap in which they found themselves, to "solve" symptomatically or maladaptively problems they experienced in coping with themselves and their situations. Each of the six persons described had decided, initially, to lose weight. Of the six, none was considered overweight at the beginning of the diet. Each did have different life conflicts to resolve and very little sense of how to resolve them.

Lonnie experienced herself as the weakest, least successful member of her family. She felt overshadowed by a physically powerful and generally successful brother and an outgoing and socially successful sister. She tried being the best behaved and the most helpful, and met others' needs constantly and desperately, only to become invisible. For Lonnie, dieting would become an achievement. She dieted as obsessively as she served members of her family. Becoming so effective at meeting the needs of others, she lost her ability to express needs of her own. Her world shrank until all that was left was control over her body weight. She had been out of earshot of others for years.

Lonnie was intimidated by instructions and deaf to guidance. The attention that her weight loss produced touched off a power struggle within her family. Lonnie was compelled by her obsession to struggle against any effort to "steal away her slimness." It was the first time Lonnie had taken a stand at odds with the will of others, and her contrariness produced a pride within her that created self-esteem where there was none before. Suddenly, she had more visibility and attention— much more. She had not anticipated this when she began dieting. This new-found attention highlighted in her own mind the dismal lack of recognition she experienced before losing weight.

Lonnie feared recovery for several reasons. First, there was the pathological fear of loss of control over her weight. The secondary gain that emerged from the illness, added attention, served to reinforce the primary pathology. Finally, Lonnie would eventually become so emaciated that her starvation would result in an organic mind syndrome manifesting increased rigidity and obsessiveness (she became afraid to drink a glass of water), and paranoia. Her self-distrust along with her failure to be able to depend on others left no lifelines toward health, only the increasingly powerful, mind-filling obsessions about thinness.

Lonnie's illness required of me as her therapist extraordinary reaching out toward her, to draw her out of her isolation. She would have to establish a bond with me, which would make her accessible enough for me to offer guidance that she could hear and not retreat from. Lonnie would experience me as a desirable competitor pitted against the safety and power offered by the illness. When Lonnie became sufficiently attached to me as her therapist, nurturing that provided safety and the authoritativeness that made me a protective person could be used to change Lonnie's behavior with regard to eating and weight, and with regard to her social role. Lonnie needed to find a way of being that was neither overly compliant nor so defiant that she had to show it by not eating. Lonnie would not engage in a power struggle with me. She would demand extraordinary nurturing. My talk would have to be protective, caring, empathic, supportive, and directive.

As Lonnie gained weight and was able to gain more insight into her feelings, she would do more of the talking. There would be setbacks during recovery. Highly stressful experiences or events would produce an increase in anorexic symptoms. Lonnie would feel like she was back where she started. The setbacks would be temporary and evolve to shorter duration and intensity. Over a period of two to three years, they would vanish. During that time, Lonnie would deal with other areas of conflict and development that would give her more effective ways of handling difficulty than resorting to anorexia nervosa.

Raphael required a therapeutic strategy different from what would be useful for the more passive anorexic. Raphael was so actively distrustful that his distrust had to be examined as it emerged. Each time he became angry inappropriately in therapy, I had to question the distrust. Ignoring it or defending against it merely encouraged retreat and resistance by Raphael. Long-term therapy with an acting-out anorexic patient requires an extraordinary degree of confronting behavior by the therapist. Raphael will still need supportive behavior, but he will also need me to prevent him from becoming chaotic.

Raphael's own expression of dependency on me will be more veiled than that of a passive patient. He will not want me to know how much he needs me. Most anorexic patients would rather not convey to their therapist how important the therapist is. While some may demonstrate clinging behavior, frequent phone calls, requests for additional sessions (all of which have to be kept in check by the therapist), others will have the same degree of attachment but are fearful lest the therapist discover this need and exploit or abandon them. The therapist should tell the patient early in the therapy that he or she will become an important person to that patient. Making the dependency explicit and defining it as appropriate reduces resistance from the first session on. For example:

Raphael looks annoyed as he enters the room.

"What's the matter?"

"I don't like being here."

"You don't like being in therapy?"

"It's not that I . . . yeah, I hate coming here. I hate the whole idea of this set-up. I hate being set apart from everyone else. I need to come here and pay you because I'm defective. You're not my friend."

"No, this isn't friendship. It's two people meeting to help one of them."

"Well, I hate that idea—that I need help."

"Why?"

"It makes me feel inferior."

"Have you ever considered how 'defective' or 'inferior' it is *not* to be capable of availing yourself of help offered to you by others?"

"It's not an achievement to be helped."

"It shows strength of character to accept help and to know when you're in need of it."

"How could *need* be strength?"

"Need *isn't* strength. The acceptance of help is a safety valve. It's flexibility. Without the capacity to accept help, you're limited to what you can do for yourself. You're excluded from taking from others and adding to who you are—in other words, growing."

"So I'm supposed to 'take' from you to grow?"

"If you're able to."

"You're saying, if I can depend upon you then I can be receptive to help from you. That means I can 'take' from you, and that helps me grow and change."

Amanda, whose bulimic anorexia is complicated by schizophrenia, presents multifaceted problems for the therapist who is developing a treatment strategy. Amanda's age (twenty-nine), however, does not alter the use of regressive techniques by the therapist. Amanda will still need to hear explanations and interpretations of her conflicts. She will plead incompetence at overcoming her problems more articulately, and a therapist would be tempted to foster greater autonomy for Amanda due to her age. This would be an error, to be met by increasingly disorganized behavior in therapy as well as intensified feelings of inadequacy between sessions. While much of Amanda's communication with her mother resulted in Amanda's feeling infantile, the mother-daughter relationship was a frightening and incapacitating state of mistrust. She had intense needs to please her mother and experienced her mother's needs as demands for Amanda to be incompetent in order to keep her mother happy and safe.

It is important to structure this therapeutic relationship so that Amanda is permitted to be dependent without feeling that the therapist is needy. This allows her to develop insight into the contrast between a healthy state of supportive dependence and her conflict-filled state of dependence intertwined with hostility for her mother, by whom she is both awed and frightened. Amanda's fears were that her mother would identify her anger and contempt, and would abandon her as punishment. This was clear in Amanda's praising her mother adamantly following virtually every statement she made that implied any dissatisfaction with their relationship. The style of the praising was desperate, as if it were more important for the therapist (and Amanda) to remember the praise than to remember the dissatisfaction. My task as therapist was to assist Amanda by stopping her from making the second, equivocating statement in each instance. For example:

"When I told my mother that I was doing an independent piece of research on eating disorders, she looked at me and said, 'Who are you to do independent research on this subject?' That really made me feel bad. Why does she think I'm incapable of research in this area? I've got more than a decade of personal experience, and I've been extremely successful in writing in the past."

"Do you feel that there are some levels of competence, in certain areas, that she's not comfortable seeing you achieve?"

"Oh, no! She's always praised my work. Even when I

was a ten year old, she praised all my schoolwork. All the awards I won she hung up on the walls of our apartment. Oh, I always felt she had nothing but praise for anything I've ever done!"

"Do you feel as if you have done the wrong thing by embarking on this research because she has expressed these doubts?"

"Oh, I don't know what I feel." Amanda gets up, walks in a circle, and goes to the mirror. "I have to see what I look like."

"Are you 'blanking' because you don't want to say anything angry about your mother?"

"Can't we talk about something else?"

"No, we have to stay with this, and you are not allowed to blank out."

She begins to cry. "My mother has always wanted me to be a success!"

"We aren't talking about your mother. We're trying to understand how you react to her. You began by complaining about a remark she made. Why don't you continue to complain in the same vein? She won't be harmed by your complaining. She's not in this room."

"But she's in my head . . . listening."

"Well, you will have to have your head to yourself then. Please resume your original complaint."

Adrienne, an adolescent acting-out bulimic anorexic, required a carefully orchestrated series of shifts in the therapist's posture. Initially, Adrienne was relieved that I understood her. She did a great deal of crying over having been misunderstood in the past, and I maintained a supportive posture. Adrienne learned to feel safe and behaved in an infantile role. When she cried it was loud, the way a baby cries. When her nose began to drip, she would sniff until a tissue was held to it; then she would blow her nose.

I had to help Adrienne make many modifications in her life as well as in her binge-vomiting state of emaciation. She had to be taken off home instruction and returned to her high school. I talked with the school authorities, and Adrienne returned to her classes where her achievement soared to its previous heights.

In sessions with Adrienne, I had to distinguish between eating behavior that deserved approval and such behavior that deserved criticism. Adrienne fought bitterly at criticism of her overeating and low weight. She now cried in objection to being criticized, because she wanted my praise. Gradually, Adrienne incorporated my values, modified her eating behavior (grudgingly), and received appropriate praise for the changed behavior. She used the accumulated praise to facilitate additional changes that also helped her avoid the criticism that so upset her. Adrienne eventually was able to predict my reactions to her, and this new set of expectations—less permissive than her parents' but consistent—became her motivation for change.

Adrienne viewed the need for change not so much as self-improvement but as a way to please me. When change was achieved, she then viewed the change in terms of positive, personal growth. The changes looming ahead, however, would be achieved more for me than for herself. As her life-style evolved, she was able to merge my ideas and goals with her own, and each new change was achieved with less stress. Restructuring eating and weight still produced the greatest stress even when her academic and social life were well organized and most gratifying. Adrienne's follow-the-leader approach on changing behavior patterns helped her break through the inertia that had kept her at a standstill for five years.

Sarah was depleted by her emaciation, and by the constant physical and psychological demands of her two small children. She, more than an adolescent, would require a highly nurturing approach. She suffered from extraordinary feelings of shame, blaming herself and labeling her uncontrollable appetite and compulsion to vomit as irresponsible. She had the least self-acceptance of the six persons discussed. From her first session, she expressed self-condemnation, none of which was of any use in helping her to relinquish her destructive pattern. It was rather the opportunity to gather support from the therapist and accept my tolerance for her behavior that enabled her to become less angry with herself. The next step was for her to learn to express appropriate anger toward others and toward situations in which she found herself that were beyond her control. Decision making about how to direct her anger led to decision making about eating and vomiting. It was the development of her own sense of will that broke the cycle.

Jeremie's fear of "rocking the boat" with her family made change difficult. She feared being abandoned by her husband and children if she risked confrontation with them. She joked in therapy sessions, spoke with friendly sarcasm, and used denial and avoidance wherever possible. My task with Jeremie was to develop a supportive relationship while using frequent confrontation—without losing Jeremie's trust or jeopardizing her sense of safety.

SOME SPECIFIC CONSIDERATIONS

Food/Weight-Related Talk   In discussing treatment of anorexia nervosa, the question frequently arises, "How much are food and eating discussed?" This varies with the patient's nutritional and general physical state. If the patient is severely malnourished and is close to medical emergency or hospitalization, it would be Pollyannaish of the therapist to avoid dealing with nutrition. Therapists who avoid the nutrition issue while treating patients approaching medical danger will reinforce the patient's use of denial. Failing to confront nutrition at this point may also imply to the patient that the therapist fears the illness and is abandoning the patient to its effects. What remains important for the therapist is not to become obsessive with the patient about eating. Casual discussions about foods the therapist enjoys eating are discouraged, because they result in the patient tempting the therapist into anorexic-like behavior, instead of the therapist helping the patient out of it. Anorexics frequently engage parents and other anorexics (if they know any) in endless discussions of food. This behavior reinforces the preoccupation with eating and enables the anorexic to avoid discussing her feelings. The patient sees herself as the leader of the discussion. In her mind she has overpowered the therapist. This causes her to feel contempt for the therapist since the therapist is seen as a person she controls, someone who has failed to remain substantial. Extorting promises from the patient to gain weight are counterproductive. The patient inevitably fails to deliver and often loses weight, to the annoyance of the therapist.

Decision Making A frequently asked question is, "How strong a role should the therapist assume in assisting the patient in her decision making?" The authoritative aspect of the therapist's posture allows for an active part in helping the patient make decisions. What must be determined is whether the decision is merely a preference or if it has significant consequences for the patient. If the decision concerns choice among ways to spend free time, the guiding principle is that free time is potential time to obsess and become anxious. The specific choices of what to do with that free time must be left to the patient. It is important to teach the patient that decisions of preference have small consequences and do not require overworking or overthinking. Decisions of consequence may be made with leadership exercised by the therapist.

One decision that commonly comes up in working with patients in their teens and twenties is which college they should attend. It is likely that they will have to remain in therapy for several years, and therapists may find themselves in the strange position of saying, "You can go to school within an hour-and-a-half travel time of this office." This is an unusually strong stand for a therapist to take, but if treatment is to continue over several years, therapy must take precedence over other college selection considerations.

Where to Live? Most anorexics in their late teens complain that their parents are too intrusive and that they would like to be free of them. It would appear that going away to a distant college would help. This, however, tends to produce an aggravation of symptoms, which later forces the patient to abandon her residential college and return home, only to find she has no way to structure her life. This dilemma can be avoided if the patient is in treatment before leaving for college. A residential college should be selected where the patient can return home easily if need be (two to three hours' distance). The anorexic living at home is often in a hostile-dependent situation. She's angry and doesn't want to eat (especially with the family), but she's frightened to be out of range of home and parents. The latter is difficult for her to admit, even in therapy. The best compromise is often for her to be away from, but accessible to, home.

Tactics in Refeeding Monitoring of the patient's weight by the therapist is advisable. The therapist should have a medical balance scale in the office and weigh the patient at the beginning of each session. If the patient's weight has dropped, she may be suffering heightened stress. If the patient's weight has risen, she is probably feeling safer and has risked gaining a bit more. When a patient sees that she has lost weight, she is relieved, although she may feign confusion or surprise to please the therapist. Her fear is that the therapist will start her on an out-of-control gaining spurt. When she sees that she has gained weight, she will become anxious and perhaps visibly upset. This may disappoint the therapist, for he may feel that the reaction is a rejection of what he is teaching the patient.

It takes time for the patient to risk gaining weight, and it is never done comfortably. The patient can expect to remain anxious, to a lessening degree, throughout the period of weight gaining. The therapist should never expect the patient to be enthusiastic about a gain in weight until weight approaches normal and the patient is free of phobic feelings about weight. The patient's weight does not have to be discussed at length, but the therapist shouldn't react with obvious enthusiasm at seeing a gain. The therapist should be supportive to the patient who has gained weight and express understanding that this has perhaps made the patient frightened. The therapist should understand that the gain is a good, though scary, event. Conversely, the therapist may interpret a loss of weight as a sign that the patient has been exceptionally tense in the past few days, then invite her to discuss this. Expressed pleasure or disappointment from the therapist over the weight change both alienate the patient and tell her she is not being understood.

THE THERAPIST'S BEHAVIOR

Behaving in a manner appropriate to the patient's needs requires constant decision making by the therapist. Nurturing interventions often involve explaining the patient to herself as well as empathic expressions of support. Authoritative interventions may range from the therapist's deciding what will be discussed to planning eating strategies, interpreting what is happening between therapist and patient at any given moment, and describing or even explicitly mapping out the therapeutic process with the patient.

The most counterproductive behaviors by the therapist would be, first, dependent communications, and, second, abandoning communications from therapist to patient. Dependent communications can be questions asked innocently by the therapist that require the patient to reassure the therapist that either the patient or the therapy is succeeding. Asking the patient if or when she will be able to gain weight is heard as a request for assurance that the therapist will be successful. Abandoning statements are those that ask the patient to assume premature autonomy. Silences, questions that ask the patient to make complex interpretations of her feelings, actions, or behaviors are examples of abandoning communications.

Both of these styles of communication are counter-productive because they replay parental behavior for most anorexics. Inferences are made by the patient that there are no substantial individuals who can help her. The anorexic withdraws from abandoning, dependent, depleted, and exhausted parental figures, including, in this instance, her therapist. And she retreats to the compelling magical system that is her illness.

13

Training the NA Therapist

Dr. B., an analytically trained psychologist, reported on his seventh NA training meeting: "For the first six meetings we've had, I've been impressed with the therapy model, but after each meeting I developed a headache. I've spent a lot of time trying to understand why this approach would give me headaches. I finally realized that you've been telling me to do what I've always wanted to do but was forbidden to do by my analytical training."

The conflict that gave Dr. B. headaches was generated by two opposing sets of ethics with regard to the therapist's behavior toward the patient. Dr. B.'s training taught him that it is his role to assist patients to fully utilize their own resources to explore, understand, and resolve problems. In this manner, patients will also come to learn that they are fully responsible for their own lives.

No one could argue with such high ideals. The issue here is

whether all people who need assistance with their emotional problems are capable of using this approach from the beginning of therapy. The active behavior that NA therapy requires runs counter to analytical training and is labeled "seductive" —offering unnecessary shelter—and "intrusive"—taking too much autonomy away from the patient. Indeed, the NA model is both of these. It has to be in order to help those who are not ready for or do not have the emotional resources for analytical psychotherapy.

Dr. B.'s conflict and his headaches disappeared after his first attempt to make use of an NA posture with an anorexic patient. He described the session:

She comes into the office and resumes her usual seat at the edge of the chair. She sits there, sort of doubled up, facing away from me. I'm feeling like a failure. I wait for her to talk and she doesn't. I get angry at her from time to time and remain silent. This time I slide my chair over to hers and talk to her about her entrance and her posture. "Ellen, I think that we should talk about how frightened you become when you enter this room. I'm concerned that it's damaging to you to stare off into space as if you were alone in the room."

She changes expression. She looks surprised and puzzled. I direct her toward me. "I would like you to try to look at me, Ellen, even though it's hard for you."

"It's not hard for me to look at people. I just don't like to."

"Isn't that the same thing? It means you're uncomfortable. We have to work toward getting you more comfortable in here."

"What's the difference?"

"The difference is that you need to become safe enough to trust me."

Now Ellen really looks confused and a bit frightened. I have never spoken to her this way, and she is also suspicious.

"I'm feeling much better about the therapy," Dr. B. concluded. "I feel like I've reached her for the first time. In the past, I've felt helpless with her, and she didn't seem to be feeling positively about our meetings either. As I feel better, she responds better, and I don't think I'm going to have a headache today."

In discussing the issue of "helplessness," Dr. B. explained, "I've always believed that it is important to be as neutral as possible in a therapy session. But I've learned to see that as an unrealistic expectation. With anorexic patients, their appearance makes it nearly impossible to be neutral or unconcerned. If I wait them out, I find that I get uncomfortable and even angry. If I talk to them and they don't respond, I feel foolish and ineffectual. After a while I can even become sleepy and daydream during a session. But the active role puts me in conflict with my training, which prohibits the therapist from behaving in a 'powerful' way. The ethical question of whether you're meeting your own or the patient's needs by behaving in an authoritative manner often comes up. Now that my patient is engaging in talk, and from what I can observe is moving out of that distant posture, I am encouraged to continue with this new approach. I do feel like a beginner with it and am aware that I will need to build a repertoire of active therapeutic behaviors and new ways of talking. I'll be doing more talking than is my pattern at this point."

Dr. B.'s conflict in starting to use an NA approach is

typical of many therapists whom I've seen in supervision. The notion of "leading the patient" raises many ethical issues in traditional as well as psychoanalytic psychotherapy.

Perhaps it would be useful here to introduce a way of viewing the emotional development of an individual who eventually becomes an anorexia nervosa victim.

OBSESSIVE-COMPULSIVE ANTECEDENTS IN THE (PRE)ANOREXIC PERSONALITY

- The (pre)anorexic experiences her parent(s) as depleted, exhausted, dependent (upon her), and insubstantial.
- She develops fear of abandonment and mistrust.
- She defends herself against these fears by becoming contemptuous and angry.
- She becomes afraid and ashamed of her feelings of contempt and anger and believes these feelings may damage insubstantial parents. She represses these feelings and becomes overpleasing, overly conscientious, even controlling with her own nurturing behavior. She vicariously enjoys the care she offers to others. She keeps her parents safe by succeeding in school. She protects them (in her mind) from worrying about her by her successes.
- She turns to external order to feel secure. She may arrange her possessions in special and exacting ways. She overworks most tasks assigned to her out of distrust of herself. Since she had experienced her parent(s) as insubstantial, she has developed little trust in them and less in herself. All decisions become crucial and are made fearfully.
- Rigidly executed rituals (inappropriate or unnecessary ways of doing things) provide a sense of safety and increase in number.

SOCIETAL PRESSURES

• Peer group pressures (much talk among today's adolescent girls is about weight and eating) combine with media pressures; fashion magazines and newspaper fashion ads all feature unrealistically, unhealthily thin actresses and models for high-achieving perfectionists to compete with.

OBSESSOGENIC EFFECT OF STARVATION AND MALNUTRITION

• Several independently developed studies show that starvation leads to obsessive thinking. (This has been observed by England's foremost expert on treating anorexia nervosa, Dr. Arthur Crisp of the University of London.)

This model interprets anorexia nervosa as a disorder resulting from societal pressures acting upon an individual with obsessive-compulsive tendencies that are in turn accelerated by the act of dieting. The longer the dieting and the greater the level of malnutrition, the more severely the obsessing is compounded by biological activity not yet fully understood.

The first areas of disturbance that the therapy must affect are the obsessive-compulsive features of the patient's personality. If the patient has experienced her parent(s) as implicitly dependent or insubstantial emotionally, the therapist must compensate for that by talking, listening, and behaving in a sensitive and substantial manner. If the patient has controlled her environment by offering care to others, the therapist needs to assist the patient in receiving care herself. The therapist also has to assist her in dealing with the feelings of helplessness that accompany the receiving of assistance. Frequent though gentle confrontations in regard to disclosure of feelings are necessary to prevent the patient from "hiding," and therefore remaining untreated, as she may have done in previous therapies.

ENCOUNTERING THE PATIENT— ESTABLISHING RAPPORT

Adolescent patients may have been brought to the therapist's office reluctantly, by their parents. The therapist may feel awkward when confronted with an "involuntary" patient. It is important to state initially that the patient's involuntary status will have to be revised by the second or third meeting if treatment is to occur. It is easiest to let the patient know she will be "taken" to therapy only once or twice, and she will have to indicate a desire to continue or the visits will terminate. This relieves the therapist of legitimate feelings of guilt about being an agent of the parents' coerciveness. It also allows the patient to "elect" the therapy into which she has been coerced. Should the prospective patient refuse to become a patient, it will be fruitless to pursue outpatient therapy.

The self-referred patient may have come voluntarily, but she is ambivalent about making herself accessible to therapy. The therapist has to become comfortable with behavior that is gently intrusive. If the patient sits passively, staring at the floor, the therapist needs to inquire about the patient's difficulty with eye contact. Lack of eye contact makes the patient unprotected, more vulnerable and alone. This can be explained to the patient. She should be encouraged but not coerced to look at the therapist occasionally. Each is equally free to see the other. The therapist must become able to foster intimacy between the two people in the room.

Therapists who in the past have viewed their role as that of a neutral witness to the patient's struggle for self-understanding will have to revise their professional self-concept to that of active leader. This quality of leadership involves energetic pursuit of the patient without communicating either dependence or anger. The semantics of nurturing become important here. The therapist must define himself or herself as an "offering" person, someone who is expert in the patient's problem. He or she must be comfortable in this role. Therapists in clinical supervision*express distress at having to assume such a posture. It runs counter to most of their previous training. This nurturing posture also threatens the esteem of the therapist. Just as many teachers feel that their esteem is most enhanced when they are teaching either bright children, older children, children of the wealthy, or cultured children, therapists often tie their esteem to the intellectually gifted patient who can "perform" by producing complex analytical interpretations with little prompting from the therapist. The therapist feels at his most adequate when doing the least talking. To some degree, the therapist must modify the idea of the kind of therapeutic behavior to which he or she attaches prestige.

BEYOND TALKING AND LISTENING

To be seen by the patient as a competent, helping person, the therapist should have some familiarity with the medical problems presented by anorexia nervosa, and some general nutritional guidelines as well. The therapist should be in touch with the patient's physician on a regular basis and be able to ask questions about the medical condition of the patient that will allow updating of the treatment plan. In this collaborative process, the therapist will learn about metabolic processes, which will enable him or her to become a knowledgeable

---

*Clinical supervision is the process by which a therapist gains professional advice and assistance from another therapist.

partner in the treatment of this psychosomatic illness. The therapist should be able to offer the medical collaborator insight into the patient's progress so that each may have the support of the other in the treatment of their patient. In this collaboration, they may share and even merge roles to some extent. The physician might do some therapeutic talking to the patient, and the therapist, with the physician's awareness, should monitor the patient's weight. Any medical concern of the therapist should be phoned to the physician for follow-up. The patient must be told that confidentiality is shared between therapist and physician. The therapist's weighing the patient also tells her that the therapist is concerned about her and, in fact, is monitoring the progress of *her* greatest concern—her weight. This, when not done in a punitive fashion, serves as a nurturing behavior. It becomes another way that the therapist takes care of the patient.

The issue of weighing the patient came up in clinical supervision with Dr. S., a male therapist with traditional analytical training, when he asked with some alarm, "Do I ask her to take her shoes off?" Dr. S. was concerned about the suggestiveness of asking a patient to remove any item of clothing—including shoes. If this is done in a matter-of-fact, discreet manner, it is seen by the patient as nothing more than the therapist's care to monitor her weight accurately. The therapist should subtract two to two-and-one-half pounds for clothing.

A gain in weight must be treated sensitively by the therapist. The patient may be upset over this and feel that she has to disguise her alarm if the therapist seems enthusiastic. The most empathic response would be, "Are you comfortable with this gain?" Similarly, upon noticing a loss in weight, the most appropriate interpretation would be as a reflection of the patient's increased anxiety. Using the scale (a medical balance scale accurate to one-quarter pound is advisable here) as an instrument of emotional as well as physical assessment lets the patient know that the therapist understands the significance of weight changes to a victim of anorexia nervosa.

THE THERAPIST EXAMINED

Proper training can help us to fill professional roles that require us to behave in a prescribed manner or posture. The posture may be formal, reserved, outgoing, appropriately warm, or firm. Nurturant-authoritative therapy requires a therapist who is or can become comfortable with the kinds of behavior that both terms connote. If one is comfortable offering care to another person and is also comfortable limiting, modifying, and remaining in an authoritative position with that person, then one can consider practicing this mode of psychotherapy. If a therapist, whether as a result of previous training or upbringing, finds this an uncomfortable posture from which to practice psychotherapy or human relations in general, it would be a difficult approach to adopt.

A nurturant-authoritative posture is similar to a parenting posture. Parents offer care and guidance and set limits for their children. The NA model is a re-parenting one. It is not recommended for all persons seeking psychotherapy, being most suitable for those suffering from anorexia nervosa, obsessive disorders, and "borderline disorders." It is not recommended, in most instances, for those persons diagnosed as schizophrenic, because they will have great difficulty seeing the boundaries inherent in psychotherapy—that is to say, they may not be able to distinguish the therapist from the parent. The model is suitable for persons who are able to understand that the relationship between therapist and patient can compensate for the missing features—trust and healthy dependence—in their development through childhood and adolescence. This should be stated explicitly to the patient.

A spoken contract to form a therapeutic relationship must be agreed upon by the two persons involved. That relationship can and should be analyzed throughout treatment. The therapist, in addition to being able to behave in a nurturing and authoritative manner, must also be able to perceive when that posture is no longer appropriate, and when a shift is required to a more conventional posture, which encourages growth, maturity, and independence. The NA posture will help the patient regress so that she may become more attached to the therapist than to the illness, and in that period of regression learn to trust herself. At some point, she is able to and needs to move forward utilizing (nervously, at first) her newly developed trust in herself. During this stage, therapeutic interventions that would have been considered abandoning or dependent become appropriate. The patient is offered, as she demands, more autonomy in the work of therapy. While it is difficult to predict length of time the NA posture is needed, it is fair to expect the patient to require it for close to two years.

While weight is an indication of the patient's becoming well, it is not the only indication, nor is it the only desirable outcome of psychotherapy. The therapist should look for a decrease in obsessiveness in general. Some anorexics displace their obsessions with food and weight onto nonfood-related objects and procedures. This would be a return to preanorexic emotional conditions and would provide for future recurrence of the anorexic modality or style. A patient has overcome the illness when she is no longer ritual-bound, is a more flexible personality, and has been able to develop mature relationships involving trust and intimacy along with the appropriate degree of interdependence. Using criteria that extend beyond eating and weight normalization protects the victim of anorexia nervosa from being abandoned by her therapist as soon as she "looks good"; they should be stated to the patient at the beginning of therapy.

Despite its manipulative appearance, NA therapy offers a more open relationship between therapist and patient because there is little that is implicit between them. The structure of the therapeutic process is redefined continually by the therapist, and there is room for the patient to argue and struggle with the therapist's point of view. The personality who develops anorexia nervosa has very little experience with confrontation, and that is built into the model. Within therapeutic limits, the relationship between therapist and patient is real. Most complaints about patients made by therapists in clinical supervision result from the therapists' difficulty in assuming an authoritative posture at appropriate moments in therapy. Dr. B. discussed with me an episode with a hospitalized patient who had been vomiting continuously, to the point of severe dehydration and potassium loss.

"I walk into her room. She is curled up on the bed in a fetal position. She is crying—no, screaming out of control. She has an IV in her left arm and a cigarette in her right hand. The amount of noise she makes intimidates me. I feel that she could vomit again at any minute. It feels like that's a weapon she could use on me. I ask her to stop crying. She screams louder. She starts gagging and I instinctively back up. She keeps it up. I finally tell her I'll come back later when she's calmer. I return an hour later and she's not crying anymore, but now she's angry at me and telling me I'm not trying to help her and I'm using her. I tell her that I can see that she's upset and frightened about being in the hospital and that if she gives it a chance, she'll calm down. At that, she starts to shout that I'm using her and I don't care about her. I leave, telling her I'll see her in three days. By now I feel discouraged and vulnerable to this kid. She shouts at me and my fantasy is that she'll vomit on me if I'm not careful.''

"Obviously, this is a patient who despite her feelings of fright can appear quite powerful. What is her relationship with her parents?''

"She seems to be very much in charge. Her mother is overly compliant out of fear that her daughter will further damage herself. Her father seems to be incapable of understanding what's wrong with his daughter. I'm not sure that he's lucid in general. He seems to go off into a daze when he and his wife come to the office for a conference.''

"It seems to me that what this girl did to you in the hospital is what she does to her parents at home.''

"Probably. Though I'm not sure what made her seem so powerful to me. I mean, she really scared me.''

"Is she physically small?''

"Yes, she's five feet.''

"Was she lying down?''

"Yes.''

"What posture were you taking physically? Were you sitting?''

"Yes. I pulled a chair up next to the bed and crouched down so that we were nearly face to face.''

"Why did you do that?''

"I wanted to convey that I was really with her.''

"Why did you want to do that?''

"So that she would perceive me as empathic.''

"When you became empathic to her chaotic state, how did you feel?"

"Terrified."

"At that point you weren't empathic, you were sympathetic. If she experiences herself as drowning, she probably wants a rescuer. When you crouched down and sat face to face with her, you were physically vulnerable, and inadvertently behaved the way her mother might have, though without the fearfulness in your voice. Then you became frightened and angry that this kid could put you in such a threatened position. At that point you walked out of the room to protect yourself from this suddenly dangerous girl."

"I didn't want to be mean to her. I wanted her to know that I was with her."

"With her *in chaos*?"

Dr. B. looks puzzled. "What's the alternative?"

"The alternative is presenting the relationship as, 'You're chaotic right now, but don't worry, I'm not chaotic, and I'll be able to help you out of your chaos.'"

"Isn't that separating from the patient, letting her feel alone, misunderstood?"

"When you saw her as a powerful person, you were misunderstanding her."

"What does one do with such an out-of-control patient?"

"Take control. You want to convey your substantiality as well as your caring. First, if the patient is lying down and crying, you stand up. You can pat her head the way you would comfort any child who was afraid of a nightmare she or he was having . . . or of living. If you are standing and she is lying down, you have avoided confusing yourself by literally drawing yourself down to her level of wretchedness. Her crying is no longer as loud to you. And you won't be frightened that she'll vomit on you, which becomes an appropriate metaphor for her overpowering and even destroying you."

"Won't I appear to be dangerous and unsympathetic to her?"

"You will appear (and really become) unafraid of her fright. You can move her out of her agitation by offering her a warm but assertive expression of calm."

"How would you do that?"

"Let's role-play this. You be Gail, and I'll play you."

(*Alternately crying and puffing on her cigarette*) "Why did you get here so late today? You don't care about me! I'm left alone in this horrible hospital day after day, and you come late. How am I supposed to trust you?" (*Screams and continues crying*)

"I can see that you're upset, Gail, but I don't believe that you think that I don't care about you." (*Standing over her and patting her head*)

"Well, you better believe it!" (*Screams again*)

(*Responding to her scream with a lowered voice*) "You're screaming and crying so loud, you just must trust me."

"You're crazy! What are you talking about?"

"If you think I don't care, why are you crying to me?"

"You're nuts!"

(*Softly*) "No, I'm not. And you're scared, and making a lot of noise so I'll know it."

Dr. B. hesitates. "I don't know what she'd say at this point."

"Do you mean that you can't imagine how she would be able to maintain her aggressive, accusing posture?"

"Yes, I guess I don't see how she could go on in that vein."

"She probably couldn't. But even if she maintained it, my responsibility is to continue to clarify which one of us is in trouble and which one is not."

"But don't you risk alienating the patient that way?"

"How?"

"You maintain such a distance. She may feel that you have no understanding of her and don't care about her."

"That's what she threatens you with. That threat manipulates you and then makes you angry with her for having overpowered you."

"Then how do you not lose the patient?"

"You keep worrying about losing the patient, and her mother keeps worrying about losing her daughter. I don't worry the way her mother worries, and she won't confuse me with her mother."

"How will she feel toward you if you strike such a tough posture?"

"I would prefer to call it a substantial posture. There's nothing that is rejecting of the patient in the posture. To answer your question, I think the patient will feel protected by me, but she won't want me to know it right away. Since she feels that all adults are insubstantial, she will want to test me to see if I'll let her down by surrendering to her moods or her illness. If I remain substantial, she'll calm down and treatment can begin. If I am manipulated by her testing, she will become disappointed with me and treatment will be put into jeopardy."

"Aren't you doing essentially what a behavior modification therapy does? It seems that you're just being a tough guy."

"A behavior modification program with no nurturing, that is, caring therapeutic component, elicits compliant behavior from the patient. If there is no attachment to another person, there is no personality change—just weight gain in order to get out of the program, the hospital, or whatever the particular setting is for the treatment. I think the problem here is that you've been the 'nice guy' and she's beaten you up. Now you're angry at her and worried about your beating her up with that anger. If she's to find you an attractive person (one to move toward so that she can move away from her hostile-dependent relationship with her parents, and her illness as well), you'll have to be sensitive to her but stronger. How do you feel about behaving in the manner we've just role-played, with your patient?"

"It feels right. When we played it out, I knew that she couldn't make me angry or make me feel threatened. I was just hoping it wouldn't make me feel like a villain. I want to try it."

Dr. B. returned the next week to say, "The shift was not comfortable for me but the change in the patient made it worth the risk. All that rage seemed to disappear. My only question is, have I only stifled her with this approach and bullied her into compliant behavior?"

"Did she suddenly become a pleasing patient?"

"No. She just calmed down."

"Are you angry with her, and does she still make you feel powerless?"

"No, actually I feel good about her at this point. I think she feels better about me."

"Her rage wasn't ventilation—the kind of anger that needs to come out. It was contempt of those who allowed her to rage on chaotically. It was behavior in search of external control by a trustworthy person."

"Well, it makes me feel better, and Gail seems calmer, so I'll continue with it. Each time I intervene in an authoritative way, it makes me a bit uncomfortable, but I'm getting used to it."

Dr. E., a female psychologist treating a bulimic anorexic woman in her late twenties, had a different problem. "I've been treating this woman for a year, and three weeks ago I suggested she lie on the couch. The patient became enraged and has been so angry that the past six sessions suggest that her continuation in therapy is in jeopardy."

"An anorexic or bulimic anorexic patient would react to a suggestion to lie on the couch and free-associate as the ultimate abandonment by the therapist. She hears you as saying, 'I have nothing to offer you. You lie down, let go of me, and work it out yourself.' She will probably continue to rage until you have her sitting up and facing you."

"If my patient is objecting to my abandoning her by putting her on the couch, how do I get her off the couch without looking like I don't know what I'm doing, and seeming insubstantial or dependent?"

"It's semantics. You simply say, 'I've thought it over and it's not good for you to be on the couch from now on.'"

"That sort of assertiveness on the part of the therapist still makes me shudder a bit."

"The model is not for the person who grew up in a

suppressive family and needs limits removed. It's for the person who has grown up with insufficient attachments to parents, and who needs both support and limits from a trustworthy person. At some point this person will outgrow her need for structure. As she incorporates the structure offered her by her therapist, she will develop nonobsessive patterns for decision making and risk taking. At that time, the style of the therapy should change to allow her to make decisions for herself."

"From beginning to end, this kind of therapy sounds like bringing up a child from toddlerhood to late adolescence."

"It's not any more original than that."

14

The Family—
Source and Resource

PRESSURES ON MOTHERS

In previous chapters, the parents of victims of anorexia nervosa have been described as depleted and exhausted. This has resulted in their being experienced as insubstantial and dependent upon the child, who eventually becomes vulnerable to developing anorexia nervosa. Yet most parents today experience themselves as somewhat depleted. How many of us find ourselves with a surplus of energy, time, money, and security?

Recent trends reveal nurturing as a low priority today to be subordinated, even for new mothers, to career planning. It seems that the prestige of being a mother has been eroded, as has esteem for the educator. We have become a society that frowns on personal care-taking and replaces it with corporate and other institutional benefits. The needy are looked down on, whether they are the poor or children. Independence and self-reliance are extolled, to a fault. Dependence is viewed as wretched and undesirable—personally, socially, and economically. These societal forces combine with the loss of prestige formerly attached to mothering, and make the mother of today demoralized as well as overworked. She is encouraged to exhort her children to become as independent as possible, as soon as possible—in many cases, before either she or her child is ready for the separation. Once the child is functioning apart from her, she is relieved of the now-demeaned status of care-taker, while at the same time she has accomplished the task of producing a successful, functioning child as quickly (and prematurely) as possible.

Several researchers* have described the relationship between mother and anorexic child as "undifferentiated" and "fused." These are terms that identify a confusion between the mother's and the child's needs. This confusion is shared by the mother and the child; they are unable to distinguish when one is meeting her own needs or taking care of the other's. This lack of differentiating causes a relationship to develop between parent and child that is riddled with guilt, anger, and overprotectiveness (by both toward each other), and characterized by mutual clinging that is devoid of trust.

Another posture acted out by mothers is oppressive-dependent, which appears to be overbearing and is in fact a defense on the mother's part that grows out of her fear of losing control of her child. The reciprocal posture to oppressive-dependence is compliant-dependent behavior. This is the overpleasing mother who is frightened of confronting her child or denying her child any request out of fear that the child will reject her.

---

*Mara Selvini Palazzoli, *Self-Starvation*. New York: Aronson, 1978.

Many mothers may be seen to act out both behaviors alternately. The result is hostile-dependent behavior by the child.

In the literature of child psychopathology, much of the responsibility for "failing to differentiate" has fallen in the lap of the mother. Her behavior is characterized as over-productive, fused, and doting, and her moods are described as anxious and depressed. What drives a mother to behave in this manner and to suffer from these feelings? A mother born and raised in Korea remarked to me, "When I saw the mothers pushing their babies in strollers, I became frightened. I had been brought up in a country where a baby is strapped to its mother's back until it can walk. There it is safe and can always hear its mother's heart beating. When the baby can walk, a mother knows it is safe to release the baby from her body. I hate these strollers but I know I'll have to get used to them." Fourteen years later her baby became a bulimic anorexic.

Mothering women have no spokesperson in today's society. Career women do. Men have the prestige of their career or the status of their income. Today's mother, then, is the most depleted and exhausted mother to date. She lacks meaningful support for her nurturing role. Will she come to depend upon the object of her nurturing—her child—as a major source of support for herself? Probably.

THE ROLE OF THE FATHER

Fathers in families of anorexics range in occupation and career from what is generally categorized as middle income (including semiskilled and skilled blue collar) through upper income, which includes medical, legal, and top corporate management positions. Within the family, the father's role is minimal with regard to the child who becomes anorexic. He is in most cases (though not all) nondemonstrative, finding it

difficult to offer physical affection, to tell his daughter that he
cares about her, that she is pretty, that he loves her. He is
uncomfortable with affection, both offered and received. He
is seen as consumed, exhausted, and often depressed by his
work. At home, he has little fun to offer his family and may
see the family as a shelter from what the outside world
expects of him. During the early child-rearing period, when
the future anorexic is one to five years of age, he will put his
greatest effort into career development, fearful that he will not
provide well for his family. While this seems appropriate, it
provides little support for his wife, who may be experiencing
his involvement in work as abandonment of her.

Father and mother have been unable to form a mutual
support system for each other. This leaves them depleted of
nurturing for each other as well as for their children.

THE CHILD

The child who senses her parents' depletion and learns how to
protect her parents with kindness and success is the vulnerable child. This child is rewarded for her success, independence, and lack of neediness. She becomes overlooked, in
time, as she demonstrates little need for attention.

Her dieting behavior begins as one more in a list of
superachievements. By the time she has outdieted all her
friends, she is trapped by her starvation's obsession-making
nature and cannot relinquish it. When she is reinforced with
attention for overdieting, she is angered by the offer of
supervision from those who never supervised her before. She
is surprised to discover that she is also pleased by the
attention. This was not her plan. She has had no authority
figures in her life (especially at home) until now and is
incapable of experiencing her parents as authorities. She
cannot stop dieting on anyone's recommendation or command

until someone can offer her the kind of security that competes with the security she has experienced from her success and perfectionism. This rigid dieting as well as ritualized behavior compensates for dependence denied to her. She feels a lack of femininity, too, due to the absence of healthy romance that should occur between father and daughter—but didn't. *Tasks* make her feel adequate, not relationships with others.

TREATMENT INVOLVING THE FAMILY

The family may facilitate recovery for the anorexic. The main consideration in deciding how deeply to involve the family in therapy is determining how resourceful the family is. If during an initial meeting parents represent themselves as overwhelmed and declare themselves incapable of change, their involvement can only be minimal. If the family system seems sturdy and parents express their desire to alter behavior, this will speed the rate of recovery. If the patient is an adolescent, the family will be asked to become auxiliary agents of therapeutic regression. That is, they will be advised to behave in a nurturant-authoritative style that augments the therapy.

COACHED BEHAVIOR

The following parenting behavior is recommended for coping with the anorexic child at home:

1. Demand less decision making from the anorexic.
2. Offer her fewer choices and less responsibility. She should not have to decide what the family eats for dinner or where to take its vacations.
3. In conflicts about decisions, parents should not retreat from their own positions out of fear their daughter will become increasingly ill.

4. A supportively confident posture should be maintained by parents when dealing with their daughter. This is *not* to suggest that harshness, rigidity, or anger be employed by parents in the maintenance of an authoritative posture.

5. Honest affection should be expressed toward the child or adolescent. Verbal and physical expression of this affection is necessary.

6. A dialogue between parents and child on personal issues *other than food and weight* should be developed.

7. Do not demand weight gain or berate your daughter for having anorexia nervosa.

8. Do not make nondifferentiating statements like, "Your illness is damaging or ruining the whole family. . . . Why did this happen to me? . . . I can't take much more of this." These statements put the anorexic in charge of the family's well-being and are received by her as dependent remarks. This throws her deeper into weight loss and illness.

9. Try to avoid abandoning statements like, "Help me to help you! . . . What can I do for you?" These statements request that the anorexic take charge of the family's behavior toward her. Since she doesn't know the answer to these questions, she feels like more of a failure. These statements are often made in frustration and even rage on the parents' part, but they should be eliminated.

10. Do not become directly involved with the child's weight once she is in therapy and under a physician's care. If you see a change in appearance that indicates weight loss, call her physician.

11. Do not demand that she eat with you, but do not allow her eating problem to dominate the family's eating schedule or use of the kitchen.

12. Do not allow her to shop for or cook for the family.

This puts her in a nurturing role and allows her to deny her own need for food by feeding others.

These recommendations will assist in restructuring the parent-child relationship from a pattern where the child takes care of or nurtures the parents and siblings while refusing nurturing from them. It also provides the family with guidelines that will prevent them from feeling helpless and enraged at their anorexic child. Family anger expressed toward the anorexic compels her to starve and lose weight, as does focusing on her illness. Most families with an anorexic child find that coping with her illness is anger provoking and frightening. They feel frustrated and powerless. It is useful for parents to engage in some kind of therapy or anorexic group-support organization in their community.

FAMILY THERAPY

Treating the entire family is advisable if the parents appear to be strong enough to adopt a nurturant-authoritative posture toward their daughter in therapy sessions. If the family seems too exhausted and each member too needy and requiring attention, it might be best to refer the parents to a separate therapist, to be seen as a couple. In that setting, they can find the support they need in order to behave appropriately toward their daughter.

PATIENT RESISTANCE TO FAMILY CHANGE

Family change threatens the anorexic as it removes her unhealthy sources of gratification. As the family declines nurturing from the anorexic and offers it to her instead, the anorexic is put into conflict. Her traditional ways of feeling adequate are diminished, and she is offered caring by those whom she dismissed long ago as incapable of it. As fewer demands are made upon her and fewer choices offered, she risks having feelings of powerlessness and being mishandled by others. She has to begin to trust, or engage in battle to reject the new system. The family may need considerable support to bear up under her resistance. Parents are also invested in the "old" system and regard their anorexic child as quite powerful; they are resistant to confronting her and are more comfortable deferring to her wishes. If the family has irresponsible eating habits, these should be revised to demonstrate eating competence. Overeaters and junk-food eaters merely serve to convince the anorexic that she is the only sane eater in the family.

Overfeeding the anorexic, or even attempting it, is dangerous, since it breaks down her trust in the family and convinces her that all everyone wants to do is fatten her up. No one in the family should be looking for a rapid gain in weight. When the patient is ready to gain weight, it should be at the rate of one to two pounds a week. A more rapid gain will tell her that she's out of control and cause her to lose the weight she has gained. She should gain weight on food she feels comfortable with—"diet," "organic," and so on.

Most adolescents and young adults maintain their weight by eating approximately fifteen calories per pound of body weight. A girl weighing one hundred pounds, depending on her level of activity, requires about fifteen hundred calories per day. As the anorexic loses weight and approaches a state of malnutrition, her metabolism slows down. Her body reacts as if she were experiencing a famine. She requires fewer calories to maintain her low weight. I have seen patients who keep meticulous calorie counts and have maintained their weight on nine to ten calories per pound. Adrienne maintained her weight of seventy pounds on six hundred and fifty calories per day. Her body temperature on a cold day would drop to 93.5°F. The body sacrifices heat and energy to survive.

If the parents are aware of their daughter's nutritional needs, they should not try desperately to overfeed her. Small portions of food separated on the plate (the way one might organize a young child's dinner) are more calming for the anorexic to face than food grouped in large, unidentifiable quantities that produce panic.

If parents can maintain a caring and calm yet assertive attitude toward their anorexic daughter, she will initially protest being treated "younger," but gradually she will experience her parents' behavior as supportive. This new family behavior will enable her to relinquish the emotional isolation that became evident as the illness developed.

15

Hospitalization

At any point in treatment, an anorexic patient may have to be hospitalized. A number of different conditions will determine whether hospitalization is necessary. The therapist should become acquainted with the patient's physician within the first few weeks of therapy. If the patient appears severely emaciated, contact with her physician should take place after the first meeting. This should be made clear to the patient. The therapist should request that her doctor evaluate her weight, vital organ functions, and vascular, cardiac, and electrolyte functioning. Therapist and physician need to agree on the point at which the patient will require hospitalization, if at all. They should contact each other regularly and be aware that the emaciated patient, out of her fear of being forced to gain weight, will try to interfere with their joint efforts in her behalf.

Both members of the therapist/physician team need to

define their roles in relation to the other. In dealing with
outpatients, both the therapist and the physician serve as
cotherapists. The physician spends less time with the patient
and emphasizes the dispensing of health information to her,
helping her interpret what a drop in weight or a drop in blood
pressure means with regard to the likelihood of hospitalization. The physician may also want to inform the patient that
she is in physical danger, but shouldn't be surprised if the
patient seems unimpressed or doesn't even believe it. The
emphasis here should be on the need for hospitalization rather
than the reality of medical danger. The fear of hospitalization
is more real to the emaciated patient than any actual threat to
her life.

The patient will attempt, in most cases, to divide the
physician and the therapist in order to protect herself from
losing the autonomy she has maintained as an outpatient. In
most instances, she has had autonomy at home and is not
used to taking direction about her eating behavior from
anyone. The idea of being hospitalized and deprived of
control over her weight is terrifying to her. In defense of her
illness and weight control, the formerly compliant patient
(and daughter) becomes engaged in an agitated struggle for
power.

The physician and therapist must agree on the specific
reasons for hospitalization and set criteria for discharge before informing the patient of their decision to hospitalize her.
If this is not done, the patient will seize the opportunity to try
to manipulate a situation where those treating her seem to be
confused. Her need to see them as confused enables her to
justify her feelings that she should not be forced to gain
weight by people who don't know what they're doing. (This
runs parallel to her need to distort her appearance and deny
that she is emaciated so that her pursuit of thinness is

justifiable to herself.) At the time of hospitalization, the two professionals must be comfortable with each other as a nurturant-authoritative team.

It is best when admission to the hospital can be anticipated by therapist, physician, and patient alike. The criterion is usually weight loss. In some instances the patient may become ill and need hospitalization urgently. This makes any kind of planning and coordination difficult; however, when the patient is confronted with graphic symptoms of illness, she doesn't engage in struggle until she feels better.

PREPARING THE FAMILY

When hospitalizing an adolescent anorexic, the therapist needs to prepare the parents in advance. They have typically become intimidated by their daughter's illness and by their daughter in general. They have learned to be afraid of directing or confronting her for fear that she will lose more weight. These are often well-founded fears. One of the most difficult—and repugnant—ideas for the family to accept is that anorexia nervosa is a severe emotional disturbance and that the anorexic is, in fact, to use a less popular term, mentally ill. Throughout their struggles with their daughter, the family still views her as "difficult," "stubborn," and "acting out to get her way."

It is very frightening for a family to accept finally that this is mental illness, an irrational state their daughter can't be talked out of. Neither threats nor bribes will make the illness go away. Failure of the family to understand this produces divisions within the family that in turn result in feelings of anger and guilt. The family atmosphere is chaotic, reinforcing the anorexic's belief that she and no one else knows what is best for her. This belief makes her resistant to therapy—and to hospitalization.

When her physician and therapist tell a patient that she needs to be in the hospital, she may ask her parents to protect her from both of them. The parents are then propelled into conflict, wishing to believe their daughter, frightened themselves of putting her in the hospital, and yet knowing she requires hospitalization. Such a series of preliminary reactions starts the hospitalization off in the worst possible way. The therapist who consults with the family and fully explains the upcoming treatment will minimize confusion.

Once hospitalization has begun, parents should visit twice a week for short periods (up to one hour). They should not bring food or attempt to feed the patient. There is no visiting during the patient's meal times. These rules help the patient distinguish between hospital and home.

PREPARING THE PATIENT

If an emaciated patient who continues to lose weight requires hospitalization, procedures ranging from admission to hyperalimentation should be explained to her, ideally before any one of them is necessary. The explanation is not given as a threat (though it is a "threat" to the illness) but as an orientation to what the patient will experience in the hospital. While the anorexic may view this care as threatening, the protective nature of hospitalization must be continually emphasized.

The therapist must not be apologetic about hospitalizing the patient. Such an attitude would be seen as dependent (on the patient to forgive the therapist) and also indicative that therapist too doesn't know what he's doing.

PREPARING THE THERAPIST

The therapist who has developed a working rapport with a patient will continue to treat that patient once she is hospitalized. A therapist in private practice, however, normally has very little to do with hospitalizations. Depending upon the therapist's training, he or she may have had some or no experience with hospitals in the past. If not a psychiatrist, the therapist may be intimidated by physicians and medical procedures. When hospitalization occurs, the therapist may inadvertently identify with the patient's fears and may feel helpless about coping with a hospital staff. The therapist, then, will need to develop an orientation to hospital structure and procedures. This should, of course, be done before the first patient must be hospitalized.

THE ROLE OF THE THERAPIST
IN THE HOSPITAL

In most cases, the therapist will be involved with a teaching hospital, one that is attached to a medical school. The physician with whom the therapist has been consulting on the case will become the patient's attending physician. This physician will supervise the routine or daily care that is administered by the interns. The interns are the physicians who will deal with the patient frequently; they will need support from the therapist on how to handle and structure the patient's routine. They will need advice on how to behave toward the patient and also need psychological information about anorexia nervosa. The therapist, then, becomes the behavioral advisor for the house staff, the residents, and the interns. In addition, the nursing staff, who must deal with the anorexic more continuously than any other group, should have access to the therapist.

The therapist should have initial meetings with the house and nursing staff to familiarize them with the patient's history as well as to coordinate behavior toward and treatment of the patient. Most therapists, in their awe of hospitals, fail to recognize the staffs' needs for support—needs that exist on every professional level—in the treatment of an anorexic patient. If the staff does not understand the anorexic's special situation, she will be treated in an uncoordinated way, and the hospital setting will only reconstruct the atmosphere of hostility that had developed within her family. The hospital staff—laypersons in treating the psychological aspects of the illness—may retaliate in anger and confusion with nasogastric feedings, threats, and punitive restrictions. The patient may gain weight to extricate herself from this punishment, only to lose the weight immediately after discharge.

STRUCTURING
THE PATIENT'S THERAPY

Hospitalization is a frightening experience for most people. The anorexic, however, doesn't feel that she needs hospitalization, and believes that the hospital's goals are in fundamental opposition to her own. This makes her more frightened than the average admission to a hospital.

If the patient has not been brought into the hospital as an emergency, and if she is not in acute need of medical care but is reaching a weight where she is at risk, several days of unstructured rest will give the staff a chance to observe her. During this time the patient can become familiar with the hospital where she may spend one to three months, or longer.

The staff must learn whether the patient is a starver or a vomiter, whether she hoards food or secretly throws it away, whether she drinks water or starves before weigh-in. They will need to observe how much walking and how much exercising she compels herself to do. They should note whether the hospitalization has resulted in her becoming agitated and manipulative, or passive and withdrawn. A primary nurse and an intern with an interest in anorexia nervosa can augment the therapist's role on a daily basis. If the therapist explains the mode of treatment to them, no one need fear the prospect of therapies that would confuse the patient. The hospital dietitian should meet with the patient on the first or second day after admission. Together they should plan menus that will allow the patient to gain a modest amount of weight—two pounds per week—so that the anorexic knows that the hospital doesn't want to fatten her up with chaotic eating.

The patient may not be able to eat sufficient quantities to maintain her weight. (A small percentage of anorexics also become too frightened of drinking adequate quantities of liquids to avert dehydration.) The patient may be designated appropriate for, and in need of, hyperalimentation. This is the surgical implantation of a small-bore catheter that is positioned in the superior vena cava (right atrium of the heart); such a procedure permits the total replacement of nutritional needs. This procedure should be explained to the patient. Initially, it is a frightening idea.

For the first time since the onset of her illness, the patient will have no control over her weight. As much as 2200 calories a day can flow through this catheter within several days of beginning the procedure. The patient can walk around, but she has to keep IV bottles as well as an infusion pump on wheels with her. She may feel desperate and think that she can't eat at all because she is already receiving so much nutrition through the central catheter. If management of the patient is handled sensitively during this period, a rational agreement should be made with the staff and the patient to the effect that she can substitute calories by mouth for the calories she is receiving intravenously. If she continues to gain weight, the flow from the catheter should be reduced until she is doing nearly all her weight gaining without the assistance of hyperalimentation.

The start of hyperalimentation precipitates a "crisis of recovery." The patient is now gaining weight fearfully and involuntarily. She is not appreciative of being rescued from death by starvation. She is often tearful and needs much support. Eating—with the support of a primary nurse, member of the house staff, or her therapist—becomes easier within a week's time. The beginning of eating is actually a tactical retreat on the patient's part since she senses the complete loss of her control over weight and wants to recover it. If the gaining and the phasing down of the intravenous fluids is handled delicately but firmly, she will retain the weight gained (four pounds, it should be noted, are lost immediately as the excess hydration is eliminated by the body). If the use of hyperalimentation is handled punitively, as a way of "teaching the patient a lesson," she will lose the weight gained after the catheter is disconnected. Helping the patient gain weight is the task, not forcing her to.

During the first days of hospitalization, the patient will attempt to alarm her family. She will want them to remove her from the hospital, where she is frightened by her lack of control over her eating. The family will need reassurance from the therapist as well as the physician that their daughter is in good hands. In her frantic attempt to retain control over eating, the anorexic often misquotes one member of the hospital staff to another. It is important that all members of the team involved in taking care of the patient speak to each other directly, to avoid misunderstandings.

Structuring the patient's eating means structuring her meals and snacks. If the patient is to give up her inner, obsessive structure, she must be offered a rational, external structure. Programming the patient's time is a problem for most medical floors. They do not have the activities offered on a psychiatric floor. When obsessive patients have nothing to do, they obsess about their weight and appearance even more than is their usual pattern. Adolescent anorexics may have their nurturing tendencies appropriately utilized on a pediatric floor by helping the younger patients.

During the weight gain, the patient will need a great deal of supportive talk from the nursing staff. The nurse should understand that each pound gained is a new terror for the patient to contend with and not the accomplishment that the nurse sees. Through this period, the therapist should see the patient twice a week or more. The patient should have more than usual telephone access to him. Members of the house staff will probably need some telephone access as well.

The bulimic anorexic presents special problems in management. Vomiting must be stopped before any eating plan can be developed. Vomiting usually stops when the bulimic enters the hospital. Lack of privacy (or even the fear of possible intrusion) inhibits many bulimics from vomiting in the hospital. Those who do stop usually stop (or substantially reduce) eating as well. They have lost their sense of satiety and fear their truly insatiable appetites. If vomiting has stopped, the bulimic can be treated like a nonbulimic anorexic patient.

To some degree, there is no appropriate setting in which to treat anorexia nervosa. If a patient is severely malnourished, she will need more medical resources than the psychiatric hospital can supply. Once hospitalized on an acute medical floor, she needs more personal attention than most acute medical patients. Often, nurses and house staff become annoyed by the special demands required of them in treating the anorexic patient. They see medical patients who are in acute distress as more worthy of their time. Any unit in a hospital treating anorexic patients should be prepared for their extraordinary illness; ideally, such a unit will have additional support persons to help in this endeavor.

Hospitals are often in need of beds. When the anorexic is out of medical danger, she is not ready to be discharged. Premature discharge results in resumption of anorexic behavior, weight loss, and readmission. At some point in the future, one hopes, halfway houses or residential treatment centers will be available for the long recovery period that many anorexics will need—a period that doesn't require intensive medical care but does require continued separation from home and family, where anorexic patterns were established. Some psychiatric hospitals focusing on adolescent patients have begun to set up specialized units to treat anorexics who are not in medical danger.

16

Support Groups

In recent years, community-based groups have sprung up to help parents and their children cope with the difficulties that anorexia nervosa poses both for the victim and her family. Often, these groups have a board of advisors consisting of physicians and mental health professionals. They are usually staffed by volunteers who include former anorexics, parents of current anorexics, and persons who have a close relative suffering from the illness. Frequently, physicians and researchers appear as guest lecturers at meetings open to the public. Such lectures are supportive, providing instructive ways of viewing this often bewildering affliction.

Most of these support groups identify themselves with the phrase, "Anorexia Nervosa Aid..." as part of their organization's name. Many of the groups hold ongoing assistance meetings for anorexics, which serve as an adjunct to individual therapy. The organizations generally do not define themselves as alternatives to psychotherapy; many will not allow members to attend meetings if they are not already in psychotherapy.

The NA therapy model presented in this book has application in the settings offered by these anorexia nervosa support groups. Following are suggested discussion topics for parents' support groups and for anorexic victims' groups. The purpose of listing these specific topics is to realign family members to produce an atmosphere where parents are comfortable behaving in a nurturant-authoritative posture that provides both safety and structure for their children. Victims of anorexia nervosa have erected protective barriers that make them inaccessible to their parents. The topics provided for the anorexics' discussion groups should assist them in relinquishing barriers that keep them emotionally isolated and ill.

PARENTS' SUPPORT GROUP TOPICS

Part I: Analyzing NA Elements in the Family

First session: Effects of the illness on the family Parents are encouraged to discuss the feelings they experienced when they first realized that their child had anorexia nervosa. They should explore how their feelings evolved as it became clear to them that this is a dangerous and chronic illness. Frustration, rage, and guilt—and the kind of parental behaviors they provoke—should be discussed. Group members should discuss any coping behavior that produced difficulties, confrontations, violence, sadness, and separation between parents and child. The connection between these conflicts and weight loss should be noted.

Second session: Caring and affection in the family system Each family has its own degree and style of verbal and physical affection. Group members should examine the quality of verbal affection (statements of caring and loving) between husband and wife. Does the couple exchange these statements often enough to feel mutually appreciated? Is there physical, as well as verbal, affection offered to their daughter? Has there always been? Was there a change at some point? Are some children easier to offer affection to than others? Does either parent have difficulty with physical affection such as hugging, kissing, and even patting on the head?

Third session: Authority in the family system Authority refers to the ability to direct members of the family appropriately in matters relating to task and scheduling, and to make decisions, large and small, that affect the family. The purpose of this meeting is to evaluate these areas: Is there authority within the family? Is that authority held by one, or both, parents? Is that authority held by one or more of the children in the family? Who makes decisions? Are they made calmly? Are they made in an agitated fashion? A violent fashion? And further, when direction is needed, is it direct—"I would like you to clean your room"? Or is the style indirect—"It's too much work for me to clean your room"? This latter statement requires the child to "rescue" the parent by cleaning her own room. Finally, how much comfort, clarity, and directness is actually operating within the family?

Fourth session: Focus within the family Every family focuses on one or some members more than others. Parents should discuss whether either one of them is the "family focus," whether it is one of their children, or whether each member of the family is self-focused, and the family doesn't focus coherently on any member.

Fifth session: Supportive caring within the family sys-

tem   Supportive caring refers to the offering of nurturing—the ability of one member of the family to reassure and comfort another member. Some areas to explore here are: Which member of the family plays this nurturing role? Does more than one member play this role? Does a child play this role with siblings, parents? Is this role played by no one in the family? If a parent plays this role, is that person comfortable with it? If it is not a comfortable role, what are the conflicts that may make it seem forced? Are openness and intimacy expressed among members of the family?

Sixth session: Rating the family structure   In terms of the preceding five topics—

1. How overwhelmed by the anorexic's illness is the family?
2. Does the family believe that the offering of care and affection is a problem?
3. Is the allocation and style of authority a problem within the family?
4. Is there a "family focus"? If so, who is it?
5. Is there a shortage of reassurance or support within the family?

Part II: Restructuring for a
More Nurturing and Authoritative Family Environment

Seventh session: Strengthening an affectionate stance   Parents who have identified problems expressing affection and caring should state specific goals they have set for improving this kind of expression among family members. Strategies should be planned for overcoming conflicts that prevent parents from offering compliments on appearance, demeanor, and likability as well as direct statements of love and appreciation to their children and to each other.

Eighth session: Redelegating authority   Parents are asked to discuss successes they are having with reassuming authority within the family. The emphasis here is on developing a rational, believable, appropriate, and acceptable authority system at home.

Ninth session: Refocusing on the children   Parents discuss problems they have in focusing on their anorexic daughter. Jealousy and anger on the part of parents and siblings can be explored. Ways of shifting attention from those who don't need it to those who do, on the basis of current need, can be shared.

Tenth session: Developing supportive behavior   Semantics and style are crucial in developing reassuring, supportive, and nurturing behavior. Role-play situations are advised here in order to help parents build a repertoire of behaviors that will make them desirable as persons to turn to for support. The overall message to learn how to communicate (and feel) here is, "I am calm. I have perspective. I can listen to you. I can help you with your problem." Messages to avoid are *hidden* cries for assistance and relief like, "If you'll just cheer up instead of ruining our day, it will be better for all of us." Or, "If you'll give us a chance, I'm sure we can help." These seem to be innocent enough remarks, but they are fraught with frustration and seem like requests for, rather than the offering of, assistance from a confident posture. As parents role-play different hypothetical situations, they can become astute at identifying dependent elements that would repel their anorexic daughter.

Parents participating in support groups using this NA model should be guided by a professional group leader, and come prepared for work—and homework—each week. The goal of the parents' support group is change in the family structure; it requires risk, exposure, and practice on the part of its members.

ANOREXICS' SUPPORT GROUP TOPICS

When assembling a group of persons who share the same problem, difficulties peculiar to that group arise. This is especially true for a group of anorexics. As they meet in the conference room, they look at each other and decide that someone else is "the thinner." There is a competitive overtone to the group. Each member wants to "cure" the others. Each wants to be the last to gain weight. It is a group of "do-gooders" who don't want to be the object of anyone else's good intentions. The most appropriate topic for such a group is competition. (If possible, bulimic anorexics should be separated from nonbulimic anorexics, because the latter may imitate the former. Often, the bulimics' ability in areas of confrontation and intimacy differ from nonbulimics.)

First session: Success, loneliness, and competition Each member is encouraged to discuss past successes in areas of schoolwork, athletics, dance, or other interests and pursuits. The satisfaction gained in success should be explored. Feelings about others one is competing with might be thoughtfully discussed. Loneliness as a factor in competition as well as an ongoing way of seeing oneself as uniquely separate from others should be examined. Dealing with the issue of competition directly with members of the group would amount to asking, "Can these eight or nine individuals really become a group?" The term *group* ought to be defined for its members. Barriers to consolidation as a group might be discussed in terms of reservations held by individual members.

Second session: Safety mechanisms Here are the ritualistic behaviors, "what we have learned to do to feel safe." This topic is best introduced by beginning with cultural superstitions and their purposes. Primitive humans tried to control the weather with the use of rain gods and sun gods. Since human beings as a species have always tried to control what they couldn't understand by theory and ritual, how do self-invented rituals differ from cultural rituals? Each member of the group should be encouraged to disclose several of her rituals. Rituals are a safety-making procedure; they guard against unknown fears. How many rituals are enough? Are food- and weight-related rituals different from others? How do they keep the anorexic safe?

Third session: History of food in our lives   Each member is urged to identify when and how weight and eating became a major issue in her life.

Fourth session: Ability to receive care   Each member is asked to discuss her comfort or discomfort with receiving advice, guidance, care, and affection. Each member's strength in offering care and support should be discussed. Why is it easier to offer care and support than to receive it?

Fifth session: Control and helplessness   When do individual members of the group feel most securely in control? When do they feel most helpless? What are some behaviors that contribute to the feeling of being in control when others are present? Do we need to be in control of others, or ourselves? The group may also discuss what helplessness means to each member.

Sixth session: Perfection, inadequacy, and self-distrust   Do members of the group rate themselves as perfectionists? What motivates perfectionism? What does it feel like to achieve less than perfection? Why are tasks often overworked? What are the signs of self-distrust? Each member should be encouraged to discuss the danger she experiences in relation to failure.

Seventh session: Confronting others and acting out on one's own body as the last arena   Group members are polled as to their ability to confront their parents. They are then polled on their comfort with confronting people outside their own families. The sharp discrepancy between the ease with which parents are confronted and the difficulty in confronting peers, teachers, and other authority figures should be explored. How does fear of confrontation lead to overcontrol of body size, weight, and bodily functions?

Eighth session: Adult roles and intimacy   Feelings and ideas about becoming or being an adult female and the role choices available to women today should be introduced for discussion. Areas for exploration might include career roles, family roles, and sexual activity. Members' ability to achieve closeness to other women, and to men (in nonromantic as well as romantic roles), can be shared.

Ninth session: Separating from parents/running back and forth   Group members might be polled with regard to their living situation. How many live alone? How many live with their parents? How many live with others their own age? How often are parents visited by those attending residential colleges, and by those with their own apartments? Is the frequency unusually high? Are members of the group clinging to home? Do they maintain childlike roles with their parents?

Tenth session: Pursuing one's "walking papers"   Here, the ability to reduce overdependency on parents, merge with peers (beginning with group members), and identify appropriate life goals can be profitably discussed.

Support groups as an adjunct to the patient's psychotherapy can provide material that will assist her in her individual recovery and growth. The structured contents of the sessions outlined deal with basic conflicts shared by victims of anorexia nervosa. The topics suggested for parents' support groups may aid the families of anorexics in developing more appropriate role structures that will also facilitate their daughters' progress. There are no sure ways to "cure" the disease, but if everyone in the patient's environment is working in the same manner to make that environment a healthier one, change will be achieved.

17

For the Afflicted

If you are afflicted, and have read this book, then you are aware that you are a victim of a disease, and not the designer of a creative way of being special. You suffer, and are condemned to defend that suffering so that you will feel powerful rather than ashamed. If you defend that suffering eloquently enough, you may be regarded as manipulative and deceitful, instead of desperate. Surely words that connote being powerful are more desirable labels than words that suggest helplessness.

In order to avoid being sentenced to living a rigidly measured existence for the rest of your life, drastic changes, which feel like great risks, are required. To make the fears that are part of change tolerable, a trusted ally is necessary. The first step, then, is to commit yourself to find a person to trust. If you construct many secret hurdles in your mind, all strangers will unknowingly trip over them. Your barriers to trust must then be lowered enough to let someone pass through, so that your solitariness can be abated. The illness, that little voice that shrieks at you from within, will then have a competitor. The voice invokes what seem to be logical objections to trusting another person. Included here are some of the catch phrases of that master of your loneliness:

You can't trust everybody.

If you don't hope, you can't get disappointed.

If you start eating, you'll never be able to stop.

You don't want to be out of control.

You've been independent all your life, why give that up now?

Most of the country is overweight and eats junk food, and you don't want to become like that, do you?

You don't feel sick. They just tell you you're sick.

Everyone is dieting, or says she should be. If you give this (disease) up, you'll be just like them.

They're all jealous of you.

They're frightened of your achievements: your thin arms, your flat stomach, your thin thighs.

They're trying to steal your thinness from you.

You have to do it yourself.

Any good demagogue always sees to it that each argument contains a shred of truth. Your error is mistaking shreds of truth for the whole truth.

An often-heard term is "achieving independence." It is sometimes applied to characterize a person's maturing and becoming self-supporting. The term *independence* remains a word that connotes virtue and wholeness. Conversely, *dependence* is a word that connotes incompleteness and potential victimization by another. In nature's model, the higher the life form, the longer the period of physical dependence by the young upon their parents. It is more difficult to evaluate the need for psychological dependence by the young upon their parents. It is far easier to determine financial and legal limits to the parent-child relationship. Achieving and completing a satisfactory period of psychological dependence means that an individual may, in times of stress, have the choice to accept the assistance of others. The option to return to dependence, relief, and support by others keeps us on balance, the way a tightrope walker performs more confidently knowing that the net is securely fastened below. Believing that there is no net below makes each step too crucial, too important, too rigid. The prematurely independent anorexic has no net below. You are ashamed of wanting nets and construct a fabric of rules, rituals, and procedures to keep you steady while walking the tightrope you live on. You always know that the fabric of that net is illusory and can't really protect you, so you continuously reweave it by adding new rituals and adhering to them more adamantly.

The solution, then, isn't to create more illusory support, but to learn how to use more real, available support. The task is to relearn a healthier dependence with another person.

Throughout the preceding pages, I have described the kinds of support that victims of anorexia nervosa need to compensate for the imaginary safety the illness offers. The victims must learn how to become patients. The patients must risk trusting and being receptive to support, guidance, care, and even affection.

The real confrontation isn't between the anorexic and the world but between the victim and her illness, that voice that shrieks those threatening ideas. You need to learn to defy that voice by trusting, hoping, and not trying to do it yourself— alone. You need to believe that you can do things moderately, that the alternative to one extreme is not the other extreme. You must come to understand that you're not in competition with everyone all the time. While it may be your differences that distinguish you from others, it is what you share with others that protects you from profound loneliness. The goal of overcoming anorexia nervosa includes overcoming all the different kinds of starvations you live with. Good luck.

Index

By the year 2000, 2 out of 3 Americans could be illiterate.

It's true.

Today, 75 million adults… about one American in three, can't read adequately. And by the year 2000, U.S. News & World Report envisions an America with a literacy rate of only 30%.

Before that America comes to be, you can stop it… by joining the fight against illiteracy today.

Call the Coalition for Literacy at toll-free **1-800-228-8813** and volunteer.

Volunteer Against Illiteracy. The only degree you need is a degree of caring.

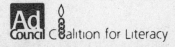

Ad Council Coalition for Literacy

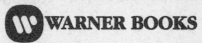